THE BEST PATIENT EXPERIENCE

THE BEST PATIENT EXPERIENCE

HELPING PHYSICIANS IMPROVE CARE, SATISFACTION, AND SCORES

BO SNYDER

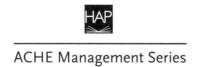

ACHE Management Series

This publication is intended to provide accurate and authoritative information in regard to the subject matter covered. It is sold, or otherwise provided, with the understanding that the publisher is not engaged in rendering professional services. If professional advice or other expert assistance is required, the services of a competent professional should be sought.

The statements and opinions contained in this book are strictly those of the author and do not represent the official positions of the American College of Healthcare Executives or the Foundation of the American College of Healthcare Executives.

20   19   18   17   16   5   4   3   2   1

Library of Congress Cataloging-in-Publication Data
Snyder, Bo (Robert M.)
   The best patient experience : helping physicians improve care,
satisfaction, and scores / Bo Snyder.
      pages cm. — (ACHE management series)
   Includes bibliographical references.
   ISBN 978-1-56793-738-1 (alk. paper)
1. Patient satisfaction. 2. Physician and patient. 3. Interpersonal
relations. 4. Medical care—Quality control. I. Title.
   R727.3.S68 2016
   610.69'6—dc23
                              2015023876

The paper used in this publication meets the minimum requirements of American National Standard for Information Sciences—Permanence of Paper for Printed Library Materials, ANSI Z39.48-1984. ∞ ™

Acquisitions editor: Tulie O'Connor; Manuscript editor: Joyce Dunne; Project manager: Andrew Baumann; Cover designer: Laurie Ingram; Layout: PerfecType

Found an error or a typo? We want to know! Please e-mail it to hapbooks@ache.org, mentioning the book's title, and put "Book Error" in the subject line.

For photocopying and copyright information, please contact Copyright Clearance Center at www.copyright.com or at (978) 750-8400.

   Health Administration Press
   A division of the Foundation of the American
      College of Healthcare Executives
   One North Franklin Street, Suite 1700
   Chicago, IL 60606–3529
   (312) 424–2800

To my wife, Jenny.

I can't believe I was lucky enough to marry the coolest lady I've ever met.

You've encouraged me to try so many things I had never considered, starting with owning a cat. Writing this book is the most recent addition to that list. A couple of great kids and other collaborations came in between.

Contents

Foreword

GIVEN THE INDUSTRY realities of growing consumerism and incentive-based reimbursement, today's healthcare leaders are asking a question that is increasingly urgent and important: "What do you do if your doctors are not getting the patient satisfaction scores they should?"

This book provides the answer—not by prescribing what physicians should do differently, but by focusing on the *leader's* role in supporting highly effective physician–patient interactions in his or her organization.

Professionals tasked with raising physicians' patient satisfaction scores include health system C-suite executives (CEOs, CMOs, COOs, and now CXOs), medical directors and vice presidents of physician services, and physician and nonphysician leaders of larger and medium-sized private practices. This book is for all of them.

Bo Snyder's work advising healthcare leaders on the Baldrige journey gives him intimate knowledge of "best practice." His book is broad and practical in the variety of resources it provides—essentially a toolbox not only of proven strategies and methods but also of checklists, scorecards, assessments, inventories, and questionnaires that can be easily adapted or used as is. It intersperses how-to information with war stories from the author and other healthcare leaders, making it an interesting and engaging read.

Our industry has a huge, unmet need in helping doctors better engage with their patients. By jumping into this challenge with both feet, healthcare leaders can improve care for patients, build financial stability for their organizations, and have more satisfied and engaged doctors.

John R. Griffith
Professor Emeritus
Department of Health Management and Policy
School of Public Health, University of Michigan, Ann Arbor

Preface

AFTER WRITING THE initial draft of this book, I was in a quandary. I wasn't sure who the target audience should be, and that was a big problem. Here's some background.

From my hands-on work shadowing and coaching physicians, it had become clear to me why some doctors perform well in their patients' eyes and have high patient satisfaction scores to prove it, and why others don't. An understanding of this dichotomy is itself valuable. But over time I became even more interested in why some clients were able to make incredible improvement, while others—even doctors who seemed eager and engaged as I coached them—were not. This became the proverbial $64 million question.

I began to work on that question by tapping knowledge from my experiences with clients, research into the science of change, and my background as a Baldrige Performance Excellence examiner and trainer and a former leader at a Baldrige Award–recipient hospital. These answers helped more of my clients improve and provided much of the material for this book.

The people who lead physicians—from department administrators and medical directors to the CEOs of health systems—have as much impact on the quality of the interactions between doctors and patients as do the doctors themselves.

And therein lies the quandary: Should this book be written for doctors or their leaders? A solution emerged with assistance from the publisher of this volume, Health Administration Press: two books. This one, then, speaks to leaders, while a later book will be intended for physicians. The book you're reading focuses mostly on (1) creating an environment that supports and requires a quality physician–patient interaction and (2) working with physicians so they can move from A to B in their personal quest for improvement.

With the purpose—helping leaders (to help their physicians to help their patients)—clarified, here's how this book is organized.

Chapter 1 begins with a brief pep talk that highlights the importance to the healthcare industry of helping physicians improve the care and caregiving they provide. It then presents a case study of a physician group that moved from mediocre to spectacular, sustained performance in patient satisfaction. Their story proves that gaining traction in a change initiative isn't rocket science, but it does require commitment and discipline.

You may notice that the group did not follow all the advice in this book. This underscores an important point: Improving does not require adherence to all my suggestions. It's more helpful to know that taking certain actions will increase your odds of success. This chapter also sets the book's practical tone. Its recommendations aren't academic; it presents only those strategies and behaviors that have proven successful for real doctors practicing today and their leaders.

Chapter 2 delves into the reasons *why* this issue is important, and why it should be important to your physicians.

Chapter 3 is a natural extension of Chapter 2, discussing how to get physicians to engage on this issue. This can be a real challenge. While some doctors have a seemingly innate understanding that the quality of their patient interactions is important, others haven't given it much thought. This chapter helps leaders approach dialogues in realistic ways that make the most impact.

Chapter 4 builds on the prior chapter with advice on how leaders can respond to the objections physicians most often make when confronted with the need to improve their interactions with patients. Often, even well-intending doctors object. Their arguments must be resolved before you can move forward.

Chapter 5 addresses my biggest frustration as a coach: Why is it that doctors who know exactly what to do, don't do it? We start with helpful concepts from the science of behavior change. Then we translate those concepts into actionable strategies that doctors can undertake—with support from their leaders—to ensure that career-long habits are altered.

The "how" of change is a difficult issue—and it's almost always overlooked. Without practical strategies for changing behavior, only the most self-motivated doctors can improve.

Chapter 6 describes ways leaders can create an environment that both requires and supports high-quality doctor–patient interactions. It offers classic insights from Jim Collins and from Baldrige Award–recipient healthcare organizations that encourage leaders to see themselves as builders of a true system for change. Chapter 6 describes the parts of a system that, once built, offers the greatest odds of high performance, and it also details the ideal tasks that leaders functioning within that system will assume.

Writing Chapter 7 was inescapable; you can't talk about patient satisfaction without discussing "the data." Some leaders are comfortable using it; others aren't. Harnessing the data—especially satisfaction data for individual providers—is crucial, but it's not without its problems. This chapter offers suggestions for dealing with the problems that perennially arise.

Chapter 8 discusses coaching as a powerful tool to help doctors discover opportunities to improve their patient interactions. It details how to shadow and coach—either personally by the reader or by building this capacity in an organization. As an external consultant and coach, I spend a significant amount of my professional time shadowing and coaching doctors as they interact with patients. This chapter sketches out a do-it-yourself approach to use when an outside coach is unnecessary or impractical.

Bo Snyder

Acknowledgments

I am indebted to Dr. Brian Tsang and Lissa Singer at First Physician Corporation (FPC), who allowed their group to serve as the case study in Chapter 1. And to everyone at FPC, thank you for your support, for wanting to be the best, and for being role models to provider groups everywhere.

Many thanks to the talented physicians, physician assistants, and nurse practitioners I've had the pleasure to coach. I've watched these masters of their craft make a huge impact on the lives of their patients—building trust and mutual respect within the time constraints demanded by our modern medical system. Just when I think I've seen every trick of the trade, one of you surprises me with something even more incredible that I can share with future clients.

I also want to acknowledge those who haven't made as much progress or are still struggling with their interactions with patients. You've prompted me to dig deeper for creative answers and look more widely for solutions. You're the reason this book is as long and—I hope—as helpful as it is.

Bill Parsons opened my eyes to *The 4 Disciplines of Execution* and leader standard work—concepts that play an important role in this book. They have helped me improve how I work with clients and changed the way I view leadership.

Don Cohen, president of Arbor Associates, has been a friend, sounding board, and source of much information over the years. His knowledge of patient satisfaction survey questions and tools is unrivaled, and his insight into ways to use survey data to improve has helped me and my clients tremendously.

Finally, I thank my wife, Jennifer Syndergaard Snyder, who was incredibly supportive at every step, beginning with, "Hey, I think you've got enough stuff here to write a book." I—and the copy editors at Health Administration Press—owe her much for her input on my early drafts.

Introduction

WHEN I STARTED helping physicians, nurse practitioners, and physician assistants (while I use "doctor" in this book, my advice applies equally to other advanced practice providers, who play a significant and important part in the care delivery team, especially as we move to value-based purchasing and accountable care) improve their patient satisfaction scores, I went looking for some practical resources I could suggest to them. I assumed I'd find a whole shelf full of useful books on how physicians can better engage and satisfy patients and earn their respect and appreciation. I was wrong.

Many articles from academic journals were impractical and too narrowly focused. And while I found some materials for the generic "caregiver"—an audience of nurses, phlebotomists, aides, and doctors too—not much literature was available for physicians specifically, or for the leaders who support them.

These two groups have unique perspectives and face unique, and increasing, challenges in the healthcare industry. Many doctors want to perform better at engaging their patients, but often they must navigate those waters alone and with little or no formal training. I can't count the times I've sat around a table with a group of physicians and heard some version of this conversation:

Dr. A: "I've never had any training in this stuff. Any of you guys?"

Dr. B: "No."

Dr. C: "Nope."

Dr. D: "Well, we spent 15 minutes on it one day in med school. But that's about it. So I guess not. No."

Meanwhile, leaders in healthcare organizations are trying to figure out how to help their doctors do better, *and* how to get physicians who know what to do, to actually do it.

Here's what happens too often:

> The leader steps before the doctors waving the most recent dismal patient satisfaction scores and implores them to do better. The doctors say they'll work on it. The leader then moves on to other pressing issues until the next batch of scores shows up three months later. No improvement. Another meeting. He again implores the doctors to improve their scores. They say they'll work on it.

This cycle can repeat itself for years, with the leaders becoming more and more frustrated and the physicians becoming increasingly irritated, defensive—or just plain numb.

The problem is that the leader is just pointing out the problem (some call this nagging), not truly engaging to solve it. He must invest some time and energy in strategies and tools to get his doctors to pay attention to the issue, support their efforts to improve, and sustain their successes.

Given the dearth of practical resources for leaders who are eager to engage with their providers and improve patient satisfaction, I decided to write this book.

I also wrote it because I love working with doctors—a privilege I've had throughout my career. I can't help with clinical issues, but my experiences observing thousands of doctor–patient interactions can help identify and fix blind spots some physicians have.

And I sympathize with leaders in organizations who work hard to support their physicians' efforts. I've walked in their shoes, so

I know the challenges they face. We all know that introducing change doesn't guarantee results. But there are proven ways to improve the odds of success.

My experiences have shown that significant improvement can be made and sustained. This book presents new insights and applies tested scientific and management principles in a new way to accelerate and sustain progress. Its goal is for patients to be better served by their doctors. Few goals in our field are as important.

CHAPTER 1

The Heat Is On: A Case Study

IN HEALTHCARE, CONVERSATIONS like these are becoming common:

Among physician leaders of a private practice: "Our group should be able to do better than 20th percentile satisfaction scores from our patients. We can't play the blame game here. It's on us. And it's embarrassing."

A hospital administrator to his contracted emergency medicine (EM) group: "We need higher patient satisfaction scores from our physicians. I'd prefer it to be with you guys, but I'm willing to switch groups if I need to."

A medical director to a confidant: "Dr. Smith's colleagues seem to respect his clinical skills, but he sure seems to rub his patients the wrong way. He's only been here six months, and he leads the place in patient complaints."

A hospitalist to a colleague: "My patient satisfaction scores are lower than most of my partners'. I'm more than a little self-conscious about it. What do they know that I don't?"

These doctors and leaders are concerned for good reason. Satisfying patients is a key to good patient care, provider satisfaction, and business success. As I expanded my consulting practice to help doctors better engage with their patients, I also started helping practice leaders and hospital administrators create environments that simultaneously support and require better physician–patient interactions.

I have looked on as some of my client-doctors flawlessly handled difficult situations, often under tight time constraints. These interactions are a thing of beauty. I've also helped open doctors' eyes to changes that immediately resonated with their patients. I've seen individual doctors and whole groups raise their patient satisfaction scores from mediocre to the 99th percentile. The personal satisfaction and professional pride they gain from this transformation is unmatched. It's gratifying to know that, over the careers of these physicians, those new behaviors will positively affect thousands of patients.

But early on, I noted that some of my clients couldn't seem to make changes and improve their scores, though they understood what they needed to do to get better and seemed motivated to improve. When I got tired of feeling irritated and disappointed in these instances, I went to work to figure out why some doctors didn't improve when others did—and how to bridge that disconnect.

I talked with my clients and researched change theory from psychology and business. I also borrowed a few insights from my experience as a Baldrige Performance Excellence examiner and from my tenure as a leader at a Malcolm Baldrige National Quality Award–recipient hospital.

In short, I became a student of the ideal physician–patient interaction and the path to get there. Over time, it became clear that successful interactions—and unsuccessful ones—have fundamental commonalities.

No, engaging patients is not rocket science. But there's a lot more to being appreciated by the patient than most people consider. Their appreciation is earned when doctors are mindful of and master specific behaviors. And I've noted again and again that physicians are most successful when their organizations create an environment that requires, supports, and recognizes high performance.

What I learned changed the way I approach my work. And my clients' success rates improved further as a result. Now I use the insights outlined in this book to help those who lead physicians make and sustain changes that their patients notice and appreciate.

No quick fix exists for turning around patient satisfaction scores from mediocre to exemplary, but the case study that follows offers proof that it doesn't have to take all that long, either, when transformation becomes a priority.

TO 99TH PERCENTILE IN PATIENT SATISFACTION: ONE GROUP'S STORY

Patient satisfaction scores can improve rapidly—not just for individual doctors but for whole groups of doctors. Take the experience of a client of mine, an emergency medicine (EM) group that made incredible progress in just one year—and has sustained it since.

The Practice

First Physician Corporation (FPC) is a privately owned physician group. It employs 11 EM physicians and 17 mid-level providers who see patients exclusively at Charlton Memorial Hospital in Fall River, Massachusetts.

Fall River is a coastal community located near the Rhode Island state line. It is predominately blue collar with a large Portuguese-speaking population. As a two-hospital town, Fall River is also served by Saint Anne's Hospital, part of the Steward Health Care System.

More than 70,000 patient visits occur each year in the Charlton Memorial emergency department (ED), with about 40 percent of those served through a fast-track urgent care model staffed by the mid-level providers—physician assistants and nurse practitioners.

FPC has always been proud of its stability and the quality of its providers. Many have been with the group for a decade or more.

FPC's Patient Satisfaction Results, Before

For years, the group focused on providing good care, efficiently delivered. It tracked the performance indicators common for EM providers: patients seen per hour, patients returning to the ED within 72 hours, admission rates, rates of mortality or transfer to the intensive care unit within 24 hours, and adherence to Centers for Medicare & Medicaid Services quality measures.

The group didn't pay much attention to patient satisfaction scores, which weren't great. That changed in 2010 when Charlton Memorial's competitor, Saint Anne's, was acquired by a new owner that soon announced a capital infusion into significant facility upgrades in the Saint Anne's ED and a strategic focus on increasing ED market share.

In no position to match the facility upgrades at Saint Anne's, the leaders at Charlton Memorial quickly zeroed in on the poor patient satisfaction scores in their ED. What had been a non-issue suddenly came into sharp focus as both a problem and an opportunity.

Charlton Memorial's senior leadership asked FPC to improve its patient satisfaction scores as a part of the broader effort to improve the scores for the ED as a whole. Much discussion ensued, both between the group and the hospital and among FPC doctors. The physicians knew they had to embrace the hospital's challenge; because the group gets paid for each patient it treats, their livelihoods were at stake.

Brian Tsang, MD, FPC president (personal communication, November 5, 2014), recalls:

My personal patient satisfaction scores were among the lowest in the group, and that helped me convince the group to accept this shift in priorities, because anything I asked them to do, I was going to have to do, too.

On this and other efforts, Dr. Tsang has worked in partnership with Lissa B. Singer, NP, MBA, CPC-I, the group's chief quality officer (personal communication, November 13, 2014). She notes:

It was important for us to show the hospital that we were in the game, committed, and serious about improvement. Patient satisfaction is just one of our improvement initiatives, but once things start moving in a positive direction, it became really hard to *not* want that continued success.

Tsang made one key request of Charlton Memorial's leaders: The hospital had to invest in obtaining a larger sampling of ED patients for its patient satisfaction survey. With a larger sampling, each provider could obtain a more convincing, and more statistically reliable, number of patient surveys each quarter, adding to the credibility and reproducibility of individual scores.

Making Decisions and Gaining Momentum

Through the spring and summer of 2012, FPC decided how to proceed. It took a while, and that patience was key to the success of the effort. Tsang says:

We're very democratic. That means things take a little more time, but the final decisions have more buy-in. And I know that the best ideas don't come from me. The group will eventually make a good decision if you let people participate and give it some time.

Exhibit 1.1: First Physician Corporation Patient Satisfaction Percentile Score, Group Composite

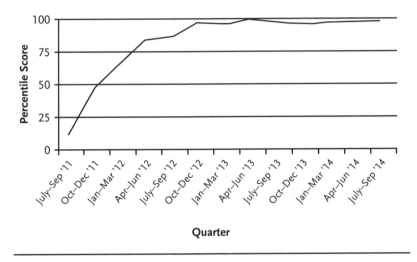

Source: First Physician Corporation and Southcoast Hospitals Group.

Interestingly, the group's patient satisfaction scores began to climb even before its first round of ideas was implemented (see Exhibit 1.1). Simply raising awareness of the issue prompted the doctors to make subtle changes in the ways they engaged with patients.

FPC started its improvement journey by providing the following educational materials to each member:

- Slides from an EM conference presentation on improving patient satisfaction
- Improvement tips from the group's patient satisfaction survey vendor
- A recent article on patient satisfaction from *Consumer Reports* that included scores from Massachusetts doctors

At the same time, it made the decision to share individual satisfaction scores with physicians on a periodic basis. Each provider received her individual patient satisfaction scores by e-mail, along with the scores of every other provider in the group. At first, the peer data were blinded; each provider knew her scores and could view the anonymous scores of everyone else in the group.

Six months later, FPC leaders unblinded individual provider names in the results. Each provider would know exactly how he stacked up against everyone else.

Rather than being fearful of exposure, the providers saw this step as a natural evolution of the information sharing that had come before. Furthermore, it caused a great deal of discussion among providers about the results and how some in the group were able to achieve higher scores. Tsang emphasizes that the scores weren't seen as measures of the providers' value as human beings but merely as another important measure of performance.

Finally, the doctors decided that the initial educational materials they received, while helpful, didn't go far enough to aid in their continued improvement. So they interviewed outside coaches who could provide one-on-one shadow coaching and facilitate group conversations about especially challenging issues.

Importantly, the group never lost sight of the big picture. The cross-town competitor was threatening the entire Charlton Memorial ED, and the FPC doctors understood their role in helping the ED improve the patient experience. Tsang says:

> We had to take ownership of what we could do to address the problem. Our ED was facing a new competitive threat. And if we didn't respond, our livelihood could be threatened.
>
> It was tempting to play the role of the victim and blame the hospital and its ED staff, who had at least as much room for improvement as our group did. We decided we had to fix our own house first. We knew that the reason patients

come to the ED is to see the doctor. If we could improve that part of the experience, overall scores for the total experience might rise, and we would have caused that to happen through our efforts.

The other benefit of making headway on our own performance is that we could show the rest of the ED team that it could be done. We could be the role model. They couldn't credibly make excuses once we had proven it could be done.

We worked with the hospital ED staff to support them and reinforce positive behaviors, but the most important thing we did was to get our own house in order.

FPC doctors began to work with ED staff on basic scripting and raising awareness. Two early examples were making sure that staff never left a patient without inquiring about his comfort and always greeting patients upon arrival with, "Welcome to Charlton Memorial Hospital. How can I help you?"

Coaching Intervention

In September 2012, I spent a week with FPC, mostly shadowing and coaching individual providers but also providing education and facilitating discussion in small groups. FPC's "naturals"— those who were born patient-interaction superstars—received minimal coaching time, perhaps one or two hours each. Most "typical" providers received two to four hours of shadowing and coaching, depending on their historical patient satisfaction scores.

I gave each provider immediate, individual feedback on his strengths and opportunities for improvement. Following these discussions, each provider identified a short list of key changes he could make to improve interactions with patients.

Some immediately began practicing their "single most important change" so I could be available to watch and provide support.

Examples of Strength Feedback Comments

"Very nice job of putting the chest pain patient at ease. He was very anxious, and you made his anxiety go away just by explaining how you were going run some tests to rule out the potentially serious causes."

"You connected with all your patients almost immediately. You greeted them all by name."

"You always paused before leaving the exam bay and asked if they had any questions or if anything was unclear. Very nice job."

"You always took a few extra seconds to share your clinical thinking with each patient. They understood the 'why' behind everything you did. They appreciated that, and as a result they had very few questions for you."

"You made a point to say good-bye to that lady as they were transporting her upstairs. She was so pleased to hear that. And she sincerely thanked you for your help."

Examples of Opportunity Feedback Comments

"When you have to leave the room for just a minute to get supplies, remember to tell the patient why you're leaving and that you'll be right back. Don't make them guess why you're leaving or how long you'll be gone."

"Always say good-bye, wish them well, and shake their hand."

"You left the room several times without asking for questions. One time the patient's family member shouted a question at you as you were leaving. Remember to pause and ask for questions before each time you leave."

(continued)

(continued from previous page)

"Slow down—especially when you first meet a patient. Give it a moment for you to build a rapport before beginning to rattle off your questions."

"Nice job with that elderly patient with many medical problems. The only suggestion I have is to pause toward the end of your interaction and summarize your main points and what's going to happen next. There were a lot of things going on with her, and I'm not sure she totally understood everything that was happening."

All received a written report summarizing key strengths, a prioritized list of change opportunities, and goals.

In the small discussion groups I facilitated, the providers took the opportunity to ask questions, learn from each other, and share personal insights. From this process, Tsang recalls:

We had to reset our thinking as emergency medicine providers. As EM doctors we like to treat critically ill patients. But most ED patients aren't very sick. In fact, most have non-life-threatening conditions, but the symptoms have made them so worried that something terrible is happening that their fear and anxiety actually become their most acute problems.

The fact is that we never thought our noncritical patients needed much of our attention. We also felt powerless to help them if they did not have a treatable acute diagnosis. Once we knew that a patient wasn't seriously ill, we mentally moved on to the next patient, hoping they might have a problem that we could actually fix.

We needed to change that mind-set. We needed to see ourselves as caring for not just a few critical patients but an entire community, and embrace the noncritical patients as just as important as anyone else. We needed to understand that even if there was no treatable emergency, these patients needed something from us, that we could provide that something, and that they would appreciate our help just as much as or more than the patient we had just resuscitated in the next room.

Our thinking matured so that we understood that satisfying our noncritical patients was not really that hard. It just required a shift in focus—away from the ABC's and critical actions and toward active listening, empathy, connection, and validation. It doesn't take that much more time, but it does require investing more of our real selves (as opposed to our doctor selves) in patient interactions. The unexpected benefit is that this approach turns potentially frustrating patient interactions into positive ones and makes the job more rewarding overall.

Post-coaching Acceleration

To maximize and leverage the impact of their investment in shadow coaching, the doctors looked for opportunities to hardwire what they had learned into their practice. One especially effective method was a quarterly "confessional," a mechanism that allowed the group to maintain a conversation on individual patient satisfaction improvement efforts over time.

This process, carried out via e-mail with lots of back and forth among the providers, involved the members articulating their key opportunities for improvement, what they were doing to improve, and what their successes were. The expectation was that everyone, even those best at interacting with patients, would identify a

Confessional Dialogues Allow Feedback and Support

Providers at First Physician Corporation used group e-mail to share progress reports about the behavior changes each was working on. Their comments* were insightful, funny, and sometimes both. Many reflect the providers being critical of themselves and their low scores. (These confessionals were generated by the group before its scores had seen much improvement.)

> *"OK, my numbers are terrible. I am not sure what happened. Most likely I reverted to my quickness, less time in room. One comment was 'minimized what happened.' So going forward I will TOTALLY empathize with the 1/4 inch cut, bump on shin, and cold × 2 days!"*

> *"I do find that explaining all the work that goes into telling a patient that it's safe to go home is typically better received than, 'Well, everything looks great!' That reassurance typically falls flat no matter how true it may be. Going through the battery of tests that were performed validates the wait and the copay. Takes some time but I think it's well worth it."*

> *"My scores suck this time around, but I don't think they are accurate! Anyhoo, I agree that people enjoy a jovial attitude at times. Also I think that buttering up the family helps the survey scores because they probably help the patient fill the survey out eventually."*

> *"My thing has been to validate the patients coming in for evaluation into the ED. I tell them that everything we have done as a cursory check in the ER was normal, but I*

*Identifying details have been omitted. (continued)

let them know that I truly believe they are having pain or are sick and that their search for a reason shouldn't end in the ER. Our job is to rule out an emergency condition that requires immediate intervention. I stress the need for them to follow up with their PCP to continue to search for an answer. Patients seem to be ok with a lack of a definitive diagnosis once I have explained our role."

"I get the patient's name before I go in, so I can address them by name from the start. I like going in without a chart in hand, but then I don't have the name unless I make a point of getting it. I already introduce myself to all family members, but I am going to start to ask them for their names, too. I have done this a few times, and I forget their names almost immediately, but they seem to appreciate it. And it helps slow me down."

"I ask if there are any questions prior to leaving the room. Sometimes I forget but go back into the room as soon as I realize this and say 'I'm sorry, but I neglected to ask if you have any questions at this time.'"

"What is working for me: letting the patient finish talking completely. Even count to five to make sure they are finished before I start asking questions. Getting water, lots of water, and box lunches. Having more fun with patients, even if they don't seem in the mood to laugh—they usually do. What I am going to try to do: try again to sit down. Drag a stool in or a trash can if necessary. Bring water for family members. Go over discharge instructions before the nurse gives them. I was good at first about thanking them for choosing us—I need to start that again. I have been printing out x-rays for fractures—that works so well that I think I will try printing even normal ones."

(continued)

(continued from previous page)

"It's hard to tell you everything I do because, honestly, I change my tactic based on the patient. I try to read my audience. Some people want humor. Some people want empathy. Some people want me to agree that the world really is out to get them and everything bad ever only happens to them. My only tactics that are consistent are: (1) Smiling. I realize that I am a smiler by nature and that others might find this difficult but I think it helps my scores. People frequently comment on how 'nice' or 'friendly' I am. . . . And I believe it's because I smile a lot. It's just a perception. (2) Giving the patient a plan. With every patient, after I get my hx and perform my PE, I tell them the plan."

"The biggest thing I try and do for every patient, especially the ones being discharged, is go back into the room and 'wrap it up,' answer any last-minute questions. Even people without a diagnosis appreciate this, at least I tried to find out what was causing the 5 years of pelvic pain."

"I do realize that I speak quickly and have incorporated a few things that have FORCED me to slow down when I speak. I have paused in the middle and at the end and admitted to them that I speak quickly and asked at least 2 times if I can clarify anything better. Since they often remember only some of what we say, this gives them a minute to digest things in smaller pieces."

"I have noticed the patient and family members in the room are shocked when you thank them for coming in. Or if I say, 'Please don't hesitate to return with any worsening symptoms or any new problems.' They appreciate that."

(continued)

"I am now working on the discharge portion of the encounter as I realized 2 or 3 times last week I discharged patients and got caught up in something and they were gone before I got back in. When appropriate (and I know already they will be going home), I will stop in as tests are coming back and say something like: 'I may not see you again before you are discharged so I'll say goodbye now. It was a pleasure meeting you. Hope you feel better soon.'"

"I have forgotten to greet the patients with their name when it is very busy, so I must get back to that. Maybe that's why my doctor courtesy score dropped. I am going to try and thank the pt. for coming to see us at the end of the visit. Maybe last impressions will revive my scores!!"

"I can honestly report to the group that I pause before starting my physical exam (and actually request permission to do so) over 90% of the time. People seem to respond well to this. It does slow me down somewhat, as I used to start examining people while I was still asking them questions."

"One thing I think is helping me is that I am less afraid to make people laugh. Even if they are really sick, it is not that hard; they are an easy audience, and laugh at pretty lame jokes. They also don't seem to be offended."

"I have taken some of your suggestions and begun addressing everybody in the room. Patients and their families seem to respond very well to this."

"I am trying to make sure I do the 'middle' visit, to give a progress report. I try to do this right after I see an x-ray or CT—then say we are just waiting for labs. I never liked going in until I was sure their symptoms had been treated

(continued)

(continued from previous page)

(nausea, pain, etc.) but too often I would forget. If I do forget, and realize everything is back but I haven't gone in yet, I will even cheat! Meaning I will go in, ask how they are, say we are still waiting for one result, then go back in 5 minutes later after I've finished the discharge paperwork to tell them the final results."

"When the ER is busy, and we are way behind, I am trying to pop in a room right next to the one I just saw to say 'still waiting on results.' The month of October, I threw it on very thick to the patients. I will be interested to see my new survey results to see if I need to completely change again or reach out for more help."

"I make a tactile gesture prior to breaking ties for this round with either a hand on the shoulder, handshake, caress of the cheek, sometimes a peck for the elderly ladies; and, of course I thank them. . . . Yeah, and what if this whole time my gentle caress of the elderly woman's face was construed as cheap flirtation by her spouse!" [Author's note: Just to be clear, this provider was having fun with his colleagues.]

"My recent scores must be wrong, I thought I was perfect? It must be a character flaw of this community." [Author's note: More fun.]

"I agree there are time limits to my smiling. It's 2:15 a.m. and it's my third back pain. The patient has had the chronic pain for months but decided to come in at this hour for repair. I used to get upset and shake my head, but

(continued)

I seem to be trending towards pulling up a chair, laughing inside, and smiling."

"Although my recent survey score is less than admirable this time around, I have tried implementing a time estimate of testing. I thought this was a good idea because it gives patients and their family a rough idea of how long they'll be in the ER. It may backfire if it takes way longer than expected, but in general, I get the sense that patients and family appreciate the time estimates. I may need to resort to carrying warm blankets if the scores don't go up next time!"

"This has made a difference with my personal job satisfaction. I find my day dominated with positive interactions and not 'me against them' type of interactions. I'm looking forward to my next round of scores. I don't know what I'll do if my scores are lower, but I'm sure one of you can prescribe me something to at least make me feel good!"

personal challenge and work on it. Providers reported on progress and moved on to other challenges once initial gains had been made. Tsang notes:

> We wanted to normalize the topic of patient satisfaction by sharing "tricks of the trade"—just like we do for technical stuff like pediatric sedation or shoulder dislocations. And we wanted to create a sense that we were all here to help each other improve.

But the process also instilled some subtle, helpful peer pressure. It reminded each provider about the one or two very important behavior changes he should be working on and encouraged follow-through and accountability to improve. It kept everyone's awareness level high and allowed the members to learn from each other.

Soon, individuals' sense of competitiveness and humor began to emerge, with providers playfully teasing and encouraging one another. About this development, Tsang says:

> We were careful to keep it constructive, but there was always some trash-talking and strutting when the scores came out. After all, we have been getting test scores for our whole lives. We had a good time with it. And it helped us to always be thinking about our interactions with patients.

Examples of the providers' confessional comments are provided in the box on pages 12–17.

Additionally, to maintain momentum and coordinate with activities in the rest of the ED, the providers began using "99th percentile" stickers and buttons. They were distributed to and worn by each FPC member, which encouraged questions from others about the group's goal to reach the 99th percentile in patient satisfaction and ensured that hospital employees were aware of the efforts of their provider group.

Soon, FPC emerged as a credible leader in patient satisfaction improvement, and it leveraged this credibility by engaging the ED nursing staff to support the efforts. For example, FPC began giving kudos to nurses who went above and beyond the call of duty with patients. In addition, staff who provided great service were entered into a drawing for an iPad tablet computer several times each year, courtesy of the group.

Patient Satisfaction Results, After: 99th Percentile

At the close of the fourth quarter of 2012, FPC had collected enough patient surveys to reveal an accurate picture of improvement. When the doctors saw that their scores had reached the 99th percentile, their pride was palpable, and their credibility within Charlton Memorial, and especially among the other members of the ED staff, was sky high. Improvement in the group's scores is shown in Exhibit 1.1, earlier in this chapter. Exhibits 1.2 and 1.3 show how individual physician scores improved.

The group immediately recognized the importance of sustaining this remarkable achievement. Today, three key approaches help its members do just that:

1. *The group monitors and reports overall patient satisfaction scores quarterly.* Any significant or sustained decrease serves as a warning to consider reinstating other approaches, such as the confessionals, which have been followed up by a mentoring program (see item 3 below). So far, scores have remained high.

2. *Unblinded, provider-specific scores are published quarterly.* Each provider is never more than three months away from having his performance revealed to peers. This mechanism makes it impossible to hide or free-ride on the efforts of colleagues.

3. *Any provider who falls below the 75th percentile in a quarter must be mentored for four hours by a high-performing peer.* Those with scores above the 90th percentile are asked to become mentors. Underperforming mentees do not get paid for their time in this session, whereas mentors are paid a bonus for their assistance. Typically, just a handful of providers are mentored each quarter, as can be seen in Exhibit 1.3.

Exhibit 1.2: 2011 First Physician Corporation Patient Satisfaction Percentile Score, by Provider

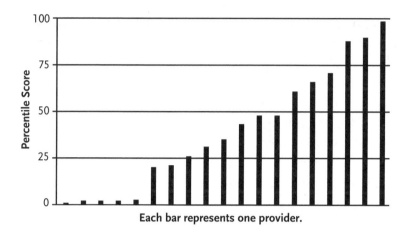

Each bar represents one provider.

Source: First Physician Corporation and Southcoast Hospitals Group.

Exhibit 1.3: 2014 First Physician Corporation Patient Satisfaction Percentile Score, by Provider

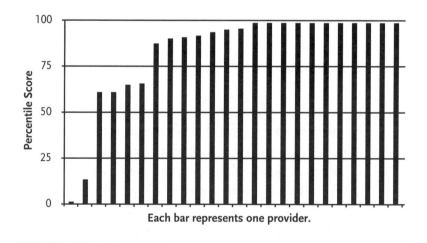

Each bar represents one provider.

Source: First Physician Corporation and Southcoast Hospitals Group.

Other Ways FPC Has Sustained Success

All providers receive any specific feedback from patients, including verbatim comments on the satisfaction survey, complaint letters, or thank-you notes. Lissa Singer says:

> When the providers hear it's me on the other end of the phone call, they immediately joke, "OK, what did I do now?" This is when you listen really well and don't say much. It is important to be empathetic. We all know the system has flaws and the patients who respond to the surveys often are not the sickest ones whom you work the hardest for.
>
> The doctors often end up coming to their own conclusions while they are venting. These calls usually end with, "Well, I know what I need to do."

Patient satisfaction performance has been built into special bonuses. When the group's mid-level providers received bonuses for serving an extraordinarily high urgent care volume in the summer of 2014, those who ranked above the 90th percentile in patient satisfaction received the largest checks. Those in the 75th to 89th percentile range received a medium bonus, and those with scores below the 75th percentile got the smallest checks.

The group did discuss adopting incentive compensation based on both productivity (patients seen per hour) and patient satisfaction scores. However, this course was soon deemed unnecessary, because the physicians moved their patient satisfaction scores to above the 90th percentile. The mid-level providers had the option to receive individual bonuses of 5 percent of their income for patient satisfaction scores above the 90th percentile, 2.5 percent above the 75th, and none below the 75th. Instead, they chose to receive a 2.5 percent bonus across the board if their entire group was rated above the 90th percentile in a given quarter, and no bonus if they were not. They wanted to "live or die together" and chose to carry their lower-scoring colleagues who brought other assets—such as being very fast—to the team. This scenario still keeps everyone on the hook for contributing to the collective 90th percentile. Each individual feels peer pressure to succeed.

The group has adopted tools for service recovery. For major issues, the retired group president, who is particularly gifted at listening to disgruntled patients, makes a personal phone contact. To address less serious issues, patients receive a "we're sorry" card that includes a coupon for a complimentary coffee and doughnut in Charlton Memorial's cafeteria.

Significantly, the group has maintained a patient call-back program throughout its journey. A nurse connects with patients in the days following discharge to make sure they have understood and followed discharge instructions and to see if they have any questions. To patients, this point of contact demonstrates the providers' continued interest in their well-being.

"How Do We Get Our Doctors to Behave Like Yours Do?"

This is the question Tsang gets when he speaks at conferences now. My answer is, help physicians find a way to practice medicine that makes patients happier *and* makes their job more satisfying.

Attitude and engagement are everything when it comes to improving patient satisfaction scores. How do we help the doctors willingly embrace the issue, identify opportunities, and make improvements? How do we help them adopt the mind-set that they aren't "good doctors" unless they interact well with patients?

In the case of FPC, the catalyst was a competitive threat. The group was mature enough to see the importance of dramatically improving patient satisfaction levels. The providers didn't ignore the problem or blame others. They sought out ways to make a meaningful impact on a significant issue.

Everyone Must Become an Owner

I'm the first to acknowledge that FPC had one significant advantage over other organizations: It is a private group with a critical mass of owners—*owners* being the important word. Ownership—whether in the literal sense (as with a private group) or in a figurative sense (as in "taking ownership")—is often the difference between placing at the 30th percentile and achieving scores in the 97th percentile.

But even if Doctor X is an employee or is not an equity owner of her group, she is still president, CEO, and chairman of the board of Dr. X, Inc. By owning her improvement, she enhances her brand, her potential success in the employment market, and—importantly—her job satisfaction.

I am frequently asked to present to physician groups on what behaviors will improve patients' perceptions of them: "Just give us the list of tips and tricks." Before accepting these invitations, I diplomatically ask whether the doctors have taken ownership of the issue so they're motivated to hear what I have to say. If not, we need to start at a different place.

Much of this book is dedicated to helping leaders help their doctors become owners in the most important sense of that word.

SUMMARY OF LESSONS LEARNED

These key points and insights from the FPC case study relate to dominant themes that appear throughout this book:

- Merely raising awareness of the issue prompted providers to begin making changes that improved their patient satisfaction scores.

- The group was thoughtful and inclusive about how to proceed, with ample input and time allowed to make decisions that had broad support. No solution was forced on the group.
- The group asked for and received a statistically reliable satisfaction survey sampling of patients for each provider each quarter.
- With some warning and a transition period, each provider's patient satisfaction data were made transparent to the others, creating a helpful peer pressure to perform.
- FPC invested in an outside coach to help both the group and its individual members. Then it made the most of the information it received from the shadow coaching experience.
- The group expects its members to achieve a threshold level of performance. If they don't, they must complete remedial work—which is unpaid. On the other hand, the highest performers become mentors and are paid extra to perform in that role.
- FPC capitalized on esprit de corps and humor among its members as they supported each other on their improvement journeys.

CHAPTER 2

A Dozen Reasons to Care About Patient Satisfaction

THE TOP-OF-MIND REASON to provide a great patient experience is that it's the right thing to do. Physicians have uniquely intimate relationships with people who are sick, scared, and vulnerable. Being respectful to them should be a no-brainer.

But sometimes it's not, and leaders can be challenged by doctors with low patient satisfaction scores who make statements such as, "I just don't think satisfaction is that important." This chapter arms those leaders with a number of go-to responses.

Certainly, how satisfied or engaged a patient is with her experience is determined by a complex set of factors, including the processes and supporting structure in the healthcare setting. However, interaction with the provider is the key driver, a concept we consider later in the chapter.

In *Practicing Excellence: A Physician's Manual to Exceptional Health Care*, author Stephen Beeson, MD, makes compelling arguments in Chapter 2, "The Case for Service" (Beeson 2006). His rationale got me thinking about the reasons—12 in all—that doctors should care deeply about the patient experience.

CLASSIC REASONS

These have been around forever, or least since medicine entered the modern era 100 years ago.

Reason 1. Bottom Line, Healthcare Really Is About Caring

You may encounter a doctor who says, "We have more important things to worry about than patients being satisfied." Is she right? No. Stellar clinical skills (one of those "more important things") aren't appreciated if the patient doesn't like his doctor's brusque questions or rushed exam. His basic expectation, that his doctor cares about him, was not met. His doctor failed, because healthcare really is about caring, and this is the best response to a physician who behaves otherwise.

Let me be direct: If a doctor isn't appreciated by the vast majority of her patients, she is not a good doctor. After all, "caring" is what the healthcare industry exists to do. It means that the physician *gives a darn*.

It really doesn't matter if a physician defines care solely as the provision of necessary services to ensure health and welfare or as a feeling of concern or interest, or both. Patients and their families expect both: skillfully provided services by someone who cares about their well-being.

Reason 2. Be Nice, or You'll Lose Them

How the physician interacts with a patient has a lot to do with whether that physician will have a chance to interact with that patient—or her neighbors, her coworkers, or those who follow her posts on social media—in the future.

Beeson (2006, 11) cites a telling finding from a Harris poll published in the *Wall Street Journal* in 2004:

> People place more importance on doctors' interpersonal skills than their medical judgment or experience . . . and doctors' failings in these areas are the overwhelming factor that drives patients to switch doctors.

A decade later, this statement is more true than ever. Take the experience of one of my client groups. Wanting to grow, it tried conducting outreach activities, advertising, joining new managed care networks, and other strategies. None made much of a difference. But when the group began to focus on delivering a great experience for its patients, it soon had a new problem: managing growth.

Volume swelled at this practice because far fewer patients left and more new patients showed up through word-of-mouth referrals, which are accelerated today by social media.

This group's approach can be likened to winning by playing a great defense, and it makes sense. We've all heard the management gurus say that the cost of acquiring a new customer is five to ten times the cost of retaining one. But the concept extends beyond economics. The foundation of patient loyalty is the relationship the patients have with their doctor. Loyal patients don't say, "I'm going see *the* doctor." They say, "I'm going to see *my* doctor."

Reason 3. Malpractice Risk Drops

Cited over and over again in the literature is the notion that a doctor's relationship with her patients has a high correlation with whether they will sue her for malpractice.

Most catastrophic medical events don't result in lawsuits. In fact, a relatively small number of doctors generate disproportionately more medical malpractice claims. But those doctors who do tend to have lower patient satisfaction scores.

Doctors who are not sued typically make an effort to partner with their patients, explain options and risks, communicate details, and make sure all questions are answered. In short, these doctors build credibility as skilled and caring people. Patients are less likely to sue individuals they appreciate and respect.

NEWER REASONS

These reasons have emerged more recently and still are in a state of flux. They relate mainly to ways publicly available patient satisfaction survey data are being used to compare healthcare providers.

Reason 4. Public Reporting Is More Metrics Based

Transparency is a beautiful thing, if your scores are good. If they're not, transparency is terrifying.

In the last decade, the Hospital Consumer Assessment of Healthcare Providers and Systems (HCAHPS, also known as the CAHPS Hospital Survey) and its sibling, the Clinician and Group Consumer Assessment of Healthcare Providers and Systems (CG-CAHPS), have empowered comparison shoppers with new sources of information.

Until a few decades ago, the patient experience was measured subjectively. And physicians didn't pay the price for patient dissatisfaction unless it caused significant and protracted word-of-mouth grousing.

No more. Objective, hospital-specific patient satisfaction data are now available for those who seek it. Since 2008, hospitals have been required to post patient satisfaction results with Hospital Compare, a public website maintained by the US Department of

Health and Human Services (www.hospitalcompare.hhs.gov), or face a financial penalty tied to Medicare reimbursement. By 2012, those patient satisfaction results became part of the Centers for Medicare & Medicaid Services' (CMS) value-based purchasing formula that rewards or penalizes hospitals.

And data availability on office-based practices is on its way. Currently, CG-CAHPS is being piloted, just as HCAHPS was a decade ago. Experts predict that CG-CAHPS results will become a factor in physician reimbursement in the near future.

The private sector is following suit, with major insurers including patient satisfaction levels in their reimbursement formulas. Expect most payment systems to include patient satisfaction as a factor in physician reimbursement in the coming years.

Reason 5. Awards Are Worth Winning and Telling Everyone About

Patient satisfaction survey vendors are beginning to wield their influence by giving awards to the highest-scoring organizations. For example, National Research Corporation (NRC 2015) recognizes the nation's top hospitals with its Consumer Choice Awards each year. NRC fields a survey of more than 270,000 households to rate the hospitals in each market. The results are published, and the top-ranking hospitals in each community often promote themselves as award winners.

Imagine a future in which the top medical groups (or, heavens, individual doctors!) in a community are recognized for their scores on private and government-sponsored satisfaction surveys. The award winners would absolutely use that information to promote themselves, leaving the others vulnerable to loss of market share.

Information companies like Healthgrades.com and RateMDs.com don't give awards, per se. But consumers now know that they can become informed on healthcare services, with just a few mouse clicks revealing past patients' comments on the quality of the doctors they are considering.

Reason 6. Value-Based Purchasing Is Here

When did hospital chief financial officers begin to care about patient satisfaction? When CMS launched its Hospital Value-Based Purchasing program, whereby a percentage of Medicare reimbursements to hospitals are put "at risk" on the basis of their clinical quality and patient satisfaction performance.

Some hospitals now receive more than they otherwise would have. Some get less. Regardless of outcome, all of them notice. Even more compelling is the thought that, for the first time, the financial impact of patient satisfaction performance can be objectively determined, at least to some degree.

It follows that the number of healthcare leaders interested in the causes of good or bad patient satisfaction performance has grown. Hospital administrators want to know how each doctor stacks up on patient satisfaction. Doctors who do an excellent job may be paid a retention bonus. Those who contribute to lower scores—or who refuse to take the issue seriously and try to improve—may be asked to seek employment elsewhere.

Reason 7. Social Media Are Present, and Growing

Never before have patients had the ability to share an unpleasant physician encounter with hundreds of friends, neighbors, and coworkers, and at lightning speed—maybe while they're still in the exam room. A single disparaging Facebook post can be devastating to a physician or practice. Patients visit the doctor when they are discouraged, angry, in pain, confused, and exhausted. It doesn't take much to push them to make their dissatisfaction known.

FIVE REASONS YOU MAY NOT HAVE CONSIDERED

Reason 8. Patient Compliance Improves

How well patients benefit from a prescribed course of treatment is directly related to how well they follow their doctors' advice. Whether taking their medications as prescribed or rehabbing correctly after a total knee replacement, their choices post-visit or post-discharge affect the clinical outcomes for which physicians are responsible.

Fortunately, doctors can influence how well patients comply. It requires demonstrating thoughtful communication, taking the time to explain clinical thinking, and outlining what could happen if recommendations aren't followed.

Taking those steps will build a stronger relationship with patients. They won't want to disappoint their doctor—a caring person whom they trust and respect—by not following instructions.

Reason 9. Power and Influence Are Solidified

Doctors carry enormous clout as highly trained professionals who are in short supply. But doctors who do their jobs in exceptional ways earn the *most* power and influence in their organizations, whether at large hospitals, group practices, or smaller physician offices. They lead by example. Their opinions are sought.

Staff listen to doctors who have high percentile scores or are known for "being great with patients." These physicians become an even more rarefied commodity than their peers.

Reason 10. Pride and Satisfaction Take Hold

This is a recurring theme among my clients. When they move the needle on their patient satisfaction scores, they're on top of the world. At work, they aren't merely applying their intellect or clinical skill set; they're making a significant impact on the lives of people who need help.

These physicians have the highest degree of satisfaction any professional could have. They respond to people in need and are often even worshipped by them. These doctors are fortunate people.

Reason 11. You Make Your Family Proud

That glow of pride and satisfaction radiates to moms and uncles and other family members:

> My son is the best doctor in the world. He is smart as a whip. But he's also a great person who has patients who rave about him. He really makes a difference.

What a great reason, all on its own.

Reason 12. Better Relationships—and Reduced Turnover—Result

Professionals who have great relationships with their customers create a positive workplace—an environment that attracts and retains other energetic, like-minded people. An atmosphere like this cuts down on the cost and upheaval of staff and provider turnover. It also nurtures collaboration—which contributes to personal satisfaction. In other words, the physicians stay happy, and their coworkers do, too.

TAKING THE NEXT STEPS

We've covered why physicians *should* care about patient satisfaction. But what if they still don't? Or what if they do care but aren't sure how to improve their scores? Chapter 3 provides insights that can inspire physicians to make patient satisfaction a priority, gain traction in the process, and move toward high percentile scores.

REFERENCES

Beeson, S. C. 2006. *Practicing Excellence: A Physician's Manual to Exceptional Health Care.* Gulf Breeze, FL: Fire Starter Publishing.

National Research Corporation. 2015 (NRC). "Consumer Choice Awards." Accessed January 24. www.nationalresearch.com/about/consumer-choice-awards.

CHAPTER 3

How to Get Physicians to Engage on Patient Satisfaction—Six Steps That Work in the Real World

THIS CHAPTER CAN help anyone who leads and coaches physicians. Maybe you work in a hospital or clinic setting and have been charged with improving patient satisfaction scores. That might mean moving a group of hospitalists from the 30th percentile to the 90th, or helping one emergency medicine doctor—who has good clinical skills but is a bit "rough around the edges"—drop from five patient complaints per month to far fewer.

Or maybe you're just trying to move the needle *any* distance in a positive direction and sustain it.

Whatever your goal, the steps in this chapter can help you get doctors fully engaged and motivated to do better.

ENGAGEMENT IS THE KEY

Until you have engagement, any effort is futile. But progress is nearly inevitable once you get a physician to buy into the effort. As Woody Allen said in *Annie Hall*, "80 percent of success is showing up."

"Showing up" in this context, however, means doctors do more than sit in meetings and agree that improving patient satisfaction is a good thing. It means they're motivated enough to assess themselves, examine ingrained work habits, and make lasting changes in how they interact with patients.

Every physician group on the planet is home to "problem personalities," varying degrees of organizational dysfunction, or issues related to internal power structures, both formal and perceived—or all of the above.

Do as I Say, Not as I Do: A Formula for Physician Disgruntlement

Physicians aren't the only ones who have to do more than just show up to improve patient satisfaction. Leaders do, too. A point of frustration I hear from physicians from time to time (and read about in their blogs) is that their managers or medical directors may nag them about low scores but don't offer any real support for helping them make meaningful changes. Physicians are also bothered when leaders fail to hold others, such as rude staff at the front desk, accountable for *their* negative impact on the patient experience. Too often, doctors feel like they are the only targets for criticism.

I empathize with physicians in this situation. Haranguing is generally ineffective, and when it goes on for a long time, it's demoralizing and irritating for everyone on the team.

So leaders, hold yourself and everyone on the team accountable for the patient experience. This shift in perspective will undoubtedly prompt you to explore new strategies, such as those in this book, and embrace a more collaborative approach. By working *with* doctors (and the front desk staff, too), you'll start to see progress.

When egged on by a humorous approach and subtle, friendly pressure from their colleagues, even the most introverted or aloof doctors *will* talk about themselves. Sometimes it's hard to get them to shut up!

Often, the ice will be broken as it was with one of my favorite ED groups. One doctor answered my opening question (which I asked lightly, looking for brave volunteers), "How do you know you're doing a good job?" with a snort and a laugh and said, "Well, obviously *I'm* not. My scores are in the toilet!" Another one chimed in, "Mine are *under* the toilet!" Their self-deprecation tore down the group's defensiveness. Eventually, even the most recalcitrant person was chiming in. Most groups have one or two doctors who can make fun of themselves. Drawing that out will aid the discussion.

Sometimes, the most productive discussion happens later, when comparative data are presented. (Sometimes if I feel like I'm pulling teeth early in the process, I will skip ahead to the data and then come back to the other steps.) I had one group of hospitalists who couldn't seem to get past complaining about their heavy work load. Discussion turned on a dime when I showed them the numbers that revealed their most productive partner also had the highest patient satisfaction scores. Often, the loudest naysayer will quiet right down when his scores are compared with his peers'.

The process for gaining physician engagement laid out in the rest of the chapter has been developed over the course of decades of work with employed and independent client groups that have vastly differing interpersonal dynamics and internal cultures. I have used it successfully with clients in a variety of specialties and in a broad range of practice settings (hospital, large group, small group, etc.). At its heart, getting physicians to engage on patient satisfaction is about personal introspection.

Focus on Accountability, Not Behavior

Recently, a colleague mentioned an article that said patients' perception of the amount of time their physician spends with them doubles if the doctor sits down during the patient visit.

Now, I happen to be a fan of doctors who sit down and look their patients in the eye. But regardless of what you or I think on the issue, is it a strategy my colleague should encourage his hospital's physicians to adopt?

I say no. Because here's the much better question: *Will establishing a specific accountability get you much, much further than giving a task-oriented directive?*

And to that I say, *always.*

Consider the result from the following scenario:

> Dr. Smith, your patient satisfaction scores are pretty low. I'd like you to begin sitting down when you meet with patients, because a recent study has shown that when a doctor sits down, the patient perceives the exchange to be twice as long as when she stands up.

First problem: How will you know whether the doctor is sitting with each patient?

More important problem: The doctor may not buy into the new behavior because she (1) didn't think of it, (2) doesn't believe it will make a difference, or (3) doesn't like sitting.

(continued)

So here you have a deadly combination: The doctor doesn't change her behavior; you don't know she hasn't changed it; and some months later you're scratching your head, wondering why Dr. Smith's scores haven't improved.

(By the way, there's another big problem in this scenario: Is the amount of time Dr. Smith spends with patients the *most important factor* in their satisfaction with her? Given Dr. Smith's style of practice, and given the particular needs of Dr. Smith's patients, they might benefit much more from a completely different change in her practice routine. If that's the case, she could do exactly as you've asked but see little improvement in her scores.)

Instead, try some nicely stated version of this:

> Dr. Smith, I'm holding you accountable for getting your patient satisfaction scores above the 60th percentile. Most of your colleagues are there already, so we know it's possible. You've got six months to do it. It's up to you how you proceed, but we'll make resources and ideas available to help you.

And sure, after the accountability is established, go ahead and make the suggestion to sit down with patients—along with other suggestions. That way, Dr. Smith has a range of behavior-changing options she can employ to reach her goal. And she is welcome to choose any configuration of those options as long as the goal is met. This approach is discussed in more detail in Chapter 5.

Sitting, standing, or doing cartwheels, you've just more than doubled your odds of getting the results you need.

THE SIX-STEP PROCESS

Step 1. Break the Ice with a Key Question

I'm a big advocate of helping doctors self-engage with some thoughtful facilitation, rather than *pushing* them to engage. I start a dialogue with physicians in a group—not individually—and I like to lead with a key question:

How do you know you're doing a good job?

In my experience, physicians give one or more of three answers:

- "I listen to my patients and treat them right."
- "I provide good clinical care to my patients."
- "I see a lot of patients every day. I'm a workhorse."

This discussion may seem elementary, but there are two reasons to have it. The first is to get the doctors to acknowledge that having patients feel good about the interaction is indeed an important part of knowing whether they're doing a good job as healthcare providers.

The second is that it gives doctors an opportunity to see you—the leader or facilitator—acknowledge that yes, other things besides patient satisfaction are important, too. You get it. You and the physicians are on the same side.

The benefit of conducting these sessions in a group has to do with the leading question. When asked individually, "How do you know you're doing a good job?" some doctors leave out "I treat my patients right." In a group, at least one doctor will bring this up. How can anyone disagree? Sometimes you can rehearse beforehand with sympathetic members of the team to prepare them to set a good example if other team members aren't as supportive.

In this meeting, you'll undoubtedly hear, "My patient satisfaction scores would be higher if I weren't so busy seeing my packed patient schedule each day." Your goal in this discussion is to make physicians see that they don't have to choose being productive *or* treating patients right. That's restrictive thinking. The reality is that today they must be productive *and* treat patients right (and practice quality medicine, etc.). This is expansive thinking used in high-performing organizations.

Step 2. Discuss Personality Types to Move from Talk to Action

Once the conversation has established that patient satisfaction is indeed an important aspect of their performance as physicians, you can discuss different types of physicians and physician personalities.

I suggest that you share a visual aid such as that shown in Exhibit 3.1—a matrix that separates doctors into groups on the basis of their clinical ability (on the *x*-axis) and interpersonal ability (on the *y*-axis). This matrix

- encourages self-reflection and group discussion of performance;
- applies humor to break the ice and soften objections;
- implicitly makes the point that there are multiple aspects of performance, and they're all important;
- introduces some structure and science to a topic that is somewhat subjective; and
- opens physicians' eyes to the fact that many different types of physicians and mind-sets come into play when providing a positive patient experience.

Let's talk about the personalities in each cell, especially the two cells in the right-hand column—those with higher clinical skills.

Exhibit 3.1: Physician Types

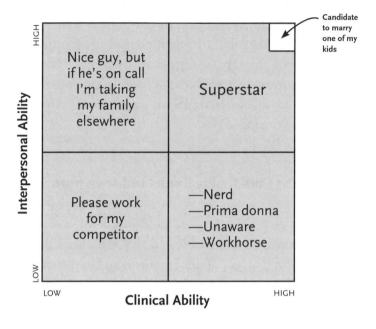

(Those in the left-hand cells are likely lost causes; in healthy organizations, those people tend to not last long.)

Superstars

Starting with the upper right-hand cell is the superstar. This individual clearly understands the patient satisfaction mandate, and patients notice. She might just be a natural at interacting with patients—in my experience, one-third to one-half of all doctors are. Or maybe she isn't a natural but recognizes what she needs to do to connect with patients, and she works her tail off to deliver. These are deliberate practitioners of the science of connecting with people.

As I've coached physicians over the years, I've noticed the following characteristics most often in superstars:

- They are self-aware.
- They are aware of how others perceive them.
- They demonstrate empathy toward others.
- They want every patient to think very highly of them and tell others what a great doctor she has.
- They want to be a high performer (and use a broad definition to define high performance).
- They are extremely coachable, hungry for feedback and insights into how to do better, and willing to do what it takes to serve the patient better.
- They seek out data that verify their performance.
- They live by the Platinum Rule: *Do unto others as they wish to be done unto them.*

Nerds

Let's shift to the lower right-hand cell. These are the doctors who don't yet fully get it. Doctors who fall into the nerd category tend to have overly developed left brains. They are the uber-scientists and brilliant thinkers who absolutely will deliver the best clinical care. But they have a blind spot for the patient's perception of them.

Prima Donnas

You know them: "Patients should feel lucky they are allowed to be cared for by the brilliance that is I." In my experience, these doctors are found in greater numbers in academic medicine, in solo practice, and in the narrower subspecialties. However, I've known some darned good neurosurgeons and cardiothoracic surgeons who are superstars. And I met one family practice physician from Iowa who was just insufferable.

The Unaware

Doctors in the unaware category often lack the sixth sense that should tell them what others need or feel—and the ability to adjust accordingly. They are often perfectly capable of interacting appropriately and well with patients but have never considered that activity to be important. Once the blinders come off, however, most improve rapidly.

Workhorses

Workhorse physicians can produce. They live for an "eat what you treat" compensation system. It's not that patient perception is unimportant to this group, it's that they feel they can make a *more* important impact by seeing more patients who need care. After all, no patient should have to wait! These doctors are trying to solve the physician undersupply issue single-handedly.

> Of course, these categories are fallible, as are all stereotypes. And note that this is by no means an exhaustive list of personality types. My clients have fun (really!) coming up with other groups to fit themselves into.

The point is to break the ice and get doctors to willingly engage in discussion, self-reflection, and sharing. Their engagement on patient satisfaction begins to deepen as each considers which archetype she fits into. Paradoxically (but perhaps not surprisingly), the superstars often think they belong in one of the other categories. These people are very self-aware and even more self-critical.

That said, most doctors belong in more than one group. A watershed moment in the discussion (and many groups will get there on their own if the facilitator is patient) occurs when the doctors discover that most of them can identify with multiple groups. Many doctors have a little nerd in them. Many also have prima donna egos—hidden better by some than by others.

At some point, it will occur to the doctors that nothing is inherently bad about any of the lower-right-hand-quadrant groups. Each doctor is who she is. Acknowledging this fact can put them at ease in identifying their personal characteristics and best approaches toward progress.

As this step in the process winds down, the physicians begin to self-assess, and meaningful engagement occurs. Once a doctor begins to "own" characteristics of one or more archetypes, he can begin to see the path toward becoming a superstar.

Step 3. Use Data to Motivate

After you've helped doctors understand that patient satisfaction is important and how their personal characteristics influence their effectiveness, it's time to show them how they stack up.

Seeing the performance data turns a philosophical discussion into a practical one very quickly. It also separates perception from reality. Other key benefits of using data include the following:

- It reinforces the efforts of high performers.
- It forces the lower performers to face reality (the data will get under their skin so you won't have to).
- It identifies role models in the group.
- It helps individual physicians begin to assess themselves using feedback from other sources.
- It introduces objectivity to the process.

Types of Data

I suggest using aggregated group data and blinded individual physician data in group meetings. Both perspectives add value, but the conversation will lack power without the individual data.

If individual data are left out of the discussion, low performers can "ride for free" on the efforts of the high performers. They can claim they are working on patient satisfaction, or worse, they can deny that they are low performers. Sharing individual data forces the low performers to own the issue.

Using aggregated data that compare the group's patient satisfaction percentile ranking against other, similar groups in the same specialty also has special power. In my experience, showing a team its performance compared to its peers can motivate like few other forces.

Typically, physicians want to be high performers. Most are competitive—they want to be the best and want others to know how good they are. There's shame in ranking substantially below one's peers. This harnessing of psychological motivators is one of the most powerful management tools available to get physicians to make changes.

Percentile rankings are especially powerful. Say, for example, a group scores at around the 20th percentile. That means four out of five other groups in their specialty perform better than they do in patient satisfaction. Ouch.

Exhibits 1.2 and 1.3 (in Chapter 1) are examples of the kind of blinded individual physician data that could be shared in a group setting. Individual doctors in the group are rank-ordered by patient satisfaction score (this could also be based on the number of patient complaints if doctor-specific patient satisfaction scores aren't available). The graphs clearly show that some doctors get it while others do not.

When to Use Unblinded Data

Calling out poor performers isn't immediately necessary. I certainly don't recommend surprising physicians in a group setting with data identified by specific doctor. However, it's fair game (and often helpful) to show the performance of individual doctors with the names blinded or coded, whereby each doctor knows her code. If you wish to increase the pressure to engage and make progress, you can tell the physicians that data will be shown unblinded in 12 months. That gives everyone a reasonable amount of time to improve her results. In our case study in Chapter 1, First Physician

Corporation unblinded its patient satisfaction results after an initial "easing in" period.

I've seen physicians rocket toward total engagement when these data are shown, especially when the group is told that support will be made available to those who desire it.

I've heard doctors, privately after the meeting, pull the leader aside and say, "I didn't know that's how I stacked up. I need to get that score up. Can you help me do it?"

I've also seen low performers raise their hands, volunteer to their colleagues that they're at the bottom of the ranking, and ask for help to move up. And I've seen their high-performing peers spontaneously offer to serve as role models and advisers. Powerful stuff.

The Elephant in the Conference Room

Often a clever doctor (usually someone who is outspoken or not afraid to point at a problem) will figure out that the overall group score can improve in two ways—either by having the lowest-ranking doctors do much better or by replacing them with doctors who are even just average.

The whole group is counting on each member to get better (or, in the case of the current top performers, to maintain their high scores). If that doesn't happen, the group may in some cases take action to improve its score by terminating poor performers (more on this later in the chapter).

What to do if

- you don't have enough surveys per doctor for statistical reliability?
- your results have multiple doctors' performance blended together?
- you don't have survey data at all?

Chapter 7 presents ways to move forward if you have any of these issues.

Step 4. Talk with Each Doctor Individually

So you've shared the data. Now you're ready for a discussion with each doctor. The goal is to merge self-reflection with the objective assessment of a leader, a trusted peer, or an objective outsider to arrive at a consensus assessment and identify where the doctor wants to be after further work.

As you talk with individual doctors, you'll begin to identify some subgroups, such as the following:

- The fully engaged (those who get it naturally or have worked very hard at it)
- The newly energized, soon-to-be-engaged (my favorite group)
- The soon-to-be-trying or pretending-to-be-trying (at the risk of getting ahead of ourselves, this is the most frustrating group because you aren't sure where they stand)
- Those to be tolerated or terminated

This last category warrants additional discussion. These are your problem children. Sometimes they must be tolerated, as when a doctor is the only provider in his specialty in your group or community, for example. Other times, these physicians are candidates for a more blunt approach from the group leaders.

The Carrot Versus the Stick

Because you're dealing with people at different levels of willingness, you'll need to consider using both reward-based and punitive approaches. From a philosophical and practical standpoint, the reward-based approach (the carrot) has much more power. But everyone should understand that punishment (the stick) is a potential consequence and may be used if necessary.

Specifically, the carrot is staying positive and getting everyone to yearn for patient satisfaction at the highest levels for all the right reasons. The carrot recognizes progress, offers resources and support for further improvement, and celebrates and communicates success.

In a group setting, I encourage using the carrot about 99 percent of the time.

When to use the stick? I advise cutting a doctor some slack if he's truly working to make progress. I give a lot of credit for sincere effort, even if progress is slow or unnoticeable right away.

But I encourage clients to be fairly unforgiving if a doctor gives only lip service—but no substantive effort—toward improvement, especially if this behavior becomes a pattern.

Step 5. When Engagement Is Not Universal and Absolute (and It Won't Be)

You've had dialogue about how the doctors know whether they're doing a good job. You've had group discussion about different types of physician personalities, and you've encouraged self-reflection. You've looked at performance data for the group as a whole and by individual doctor.

But full engagement among all the group's members just isn't there.

Don't worry. This is almost always the case. Regardless of what the physicians tell you, some will not engage. Sometimes, most of the group will be in a funk. How can you get them unstuck? What can you do when your doctors' engagement level is less than ideal?

Start by Working with Those Who Are Willing

People who treat alcoholics will tell you that those who voluntarily attend Alcoholics Anonymous meetings tend to manage their disease much better than those who go because the court orders them to. Work with your doctors who either volunteer *for* help or volunteer *to* help. You can deal with the chronically unengaged later.

Make your superstars your leaders and ambassadors. Ask them to be patient satisfaction role models for the group. Share their data as examples of what can be achieved. Encourage your less patient-friendly doctors to seek them out as coaches and mentors.

Some of your superstars will still have room for improvement. Work with the "already pretty good" doctors to raise their scores from, say, the 75th percentile to the 95th percentile. Fast improvement is often possible with this group. A key component of this effort is to make sure everyone knows exactly what skills the individuals in this group are working on. The superstars will prove that improvement can occur even among those who were doing fairly well already. From there, group momentum will build, and others will be encouraged to engage.

Now identify the doctors who were unaware at the beginning of the process but have the capacity to do much better. Offer support and coaching to raise them from, for example, the 20th percentile to the 80th percentile.

This is my favorite group to work with because of its potential for rapid improvement. Members of this category are your soon-to-be superstars. Noticeable effort from this group and indications of their performance improvement send a strong message to those who aren't engaged. Chances are good that new leaders will emerge to build even more momentum for the group.

Use Reciprocity to Get the Team Unstuck

As mentioned earlier, sometimes a whole group will bog down, nurse a bad attitude, and seem unable to move forward. If that happens, it's usually beneficial to take a step back, stay positive, and start building a relationship of reciprocity.

This can take some time.

The concept is simple. It is based on a symbiotic relationship in which each party benefits by living up to its end of a bargain: "I do something nice for you. You do something nice for me." (See the following box for an example.)

The Power of Reciprocity

"We've got to get the docs to . . . ."

How many times have you heard that? Said that?

For my entire career in healthcare—27 years and counting—engaging doctors has appeared on the top ten list of "Things Healthcare Executives Wish They Could Do Better."

As organizations work to improve care delivery, physicians are often key partners in moving the organization forward. They are busy, powerful people. Many are also cooperative, but all of them have a mountain of priorities to address in their personal and professional lives. How can you get them to put your issue on their dance card?

Answer Their (Usually) Unspoken Question, "What's in It for Me?"

I learned this strategy the hard way earlier in my career, when I was administrator of orthopedic services. We had a big problem with the cost of implants. We needed the surgeons to agree to work with fewer manufacturers in exchange for a price discount that would bring our implant business back into the black.

So we called a meeting with our orthopods to discuss it. You know—at 6:30 a.m., before cases start at 7:30. The only surgeon who showed up was the medical director, because he had to.

We were sure there must have been some miscommunication, so we tried again a few months later. No one showed up.

(continued)

(continued from previous page)

So we reached out to a few of the surgeons to ask why. The answer was clear: They were too busy doing other stuff they deemed more important. They weren't unsympathetic to our issue, but they had "higher value" things going on those mornings.

So, we tried a third time—except this time, we announced the meeting as the "Asking the Surgeons What Issues with Our Orthopedic Program Drive Them Nuts So We Can Fix Them" meeting.

The result? Standing-room-only participation.

We asked the doctors to prioritize their problems with the hospital, and we started working on their top concerns. We met every three months for progress updates. After nine months (I didn't say this was a quick process), the hospital had solved problems that had been thorns for the doctors forever.

The surgeons were appreciative. And *after* we had established this track record of taking their issues seriously, we asked, "Can you help us with the implant cost problem?" And they said, "Sure, let's put it on our next quarterly meeting agenda." And we did.

The key is: At that point, how could they say "no"?

We had established reciprocity. We were working hard on the physicians' biggest concerns and making progress. So they were ready to help us. As a result, after another six months of work, we reduced our implant vendors to two in exchange for price discounts that turned red ink to black. All accomplished with surgeon support. *(continued)*

By the way, after this initiative, the group began to move mountains. Several years later we had become such a good place for orthopedic surgeons to work that we had grown market share from 40 percent to 60 percent.

Reciprocity makes most things possible. In my opinion, it *tops* the top ten list of "Tools Healthcare Executives Should Use to Get Doctors to Engage."

Start by focusing on one broad issue that the physician group would love to have addressed. For example: "Yes, doctors, we understand that our turnaround time for diagnostic testing results is too long and leads to dissatisfied patients. And we're going to work hard on that."

Then actually make headway on that issue. And this may take months and months.

Once progress has been made on the doctors' concern, you've built credibility and trust. They owe you one. And the thing they owe you might be working on their patient satisfaction scores.

If you're trying to gain physicians' engagement on the issue of patient satisfaction scores—or anything else—you have to show them what's in it for them, or at the very least show them what your organization is doing beyond pointing fingers at doctors. Because there are always many things that organizations can do to improve the patient experience, and credibility with the doctors will expand greatly if you are working on some of those things.

Then you will have established a relationship based on reciprocity—a near-magical state of being (and I am not overstating this) in which parties have seen the importance of moving forward and improving by addressing mutual concerns.

Step 6. If You Have To, Haul Out the Stick

In my experience, the hardest thing to do is sort out the soon-to-be-trying from the pretending-to-try doctors. Sometimes, making this differentiation can take years. Most doctors won't say they refuse to improve patient satisfaction. They may talk a good story, but their scores don't budge.

At some point, you need to take action—get out the stick. When you use "stick" approaches, you must be prepared for the doctor to leave—and by this time, separation may be a good solution. I understand that physicians bring necessary skills to a healthcare organization and are in short supply. But don't let them roll over you. At least weigh the possibility of letting one go.

In fact, I would argue that *you are not really serious about patient satisfaction unless you're willing to part ways with a few doctors over the issue.* Leaders who have been willing to take this action have experienced a renewed sense of confidence afterward, and the impact on the remaining group is usually very positive—just as positive as if they had removed a doctor who was widely recognized as having poor clinical judgment.

Some Stick Approaches

- Share individual physicians' patient satisfaction performance data with the whole group with the names of the doctors *unblinded.* If your measurement tool is sophisticated enough, it's possible to show the group what would happen to the group's overall score if the few lowest performers were removed. Uncomfortable? Absolutely. Effective? Often.
- Include patient satisfaction as a significant consideration in awarding bonuses.

- Alter policies so that individual patient satisfaction performance is factored into awarding vacation and shift preferences. High performers get their first choice.
- Sever employment of the doctor. Termination sends a strong message to others who aren't fully engaged. And chances are good that the replacement will be a stronger performer.

Remember, at this point, you will have been talking about the importance of patient satisfaction for months, if not years. If a low-performing physician is upset at losing her preferred vacation week, for example, tell her, "This should not surprise you at all. We've been working toward accountability on this topic for a long, long time."

Former football coach Lou Holtz was once asked how he motivated his team. His answer was that motivation is simple: You get rid of those who are not motivated. Coach Holtz knew that cutting low performers raises the average of those remaining team members *and* tends to motivate those members to increase their efforts. The team and its results—which reflect the experience of *all your patients*, remember—should be more important than any single physician.

CHAPTER 4

Dealing with the Objections of Skeptical Physicians

SOME DOCTORS REFLEXIVELY object when I suggest ways they can improve their interactions with patients. Self-reflection and change are hard, especially if your typical day is spent on roller skates. That's just human nature.

I've found that arguing with physicians does little good. And it's a good thing the key is not winning the argument. Instead, try to lead doctors toward embracing a new point of view. Read on, and trust me that this can be done.

TYPICAL OBJECTIONS

I'm Already Doing Just Fine

Often this objection is unspoken, but it's there, just the same. When I shadow physicians, I find that between one-third and one-half of them really *do* handle interactions with their patients well.

But others focus too much on "getting the job done," whether that's providing good clinical quality or seeing an enormous case-load. They often lack self-awareness and don't try to understand and meet the individual needs of each patient. These physicians must redefine "doing fine."

- Given that most patients won't tell you if they're dissatisfied, how do you know you're doing fine?
- Do your patient satisfaction scores support your assessment? What about patient complaints?
- Do the nurses or your medical assistant rave about your bedside manner?
- Have you invited an impartial person to observe your interactions and offer an assessment and some feedback? (Staff and colleagues know which doctors interact well with patients but may be uncomfortable giving negative feedback. So you need either performance data, such as survey results, or an assessment by an objective third party. See Chapter 5 for a staff feedback questionnaire or Chapter 8 on do-it-yourself shadow coaching.)

My Productivity Will Suffer

Physicians often assume that the magic answer to better patient engagement is to spend more time with each patient. The problem is, in their mind, they don't know where they can find that time. To be fair, they often can't.

Responses

- Most groups have highly productive doctors who also have good patient satisfaction scores. They've figured out a way to make it work, and we can, too.
- We keep score differently now. We no longer choose maximizing productivity *or* patient satisfaction. The new realities in healthcare require us to focus on productivity *and* patient satisfaction. And of course, the expectation to deliver on the technical aspects of quality care is a given.

- (If the genesis of this objection is the impact productivity has on physician income:) In our industry's new reality, patient satisfaction is one of the factors already affecting income, or it will be soon.
- If improved productivity is our goal, we can achieve it without depriving patients of time spent with you. Time with their physician is what they deserve.
- There are ways to improve the physician–patient interaction without spending more time with them. (My forthcoming book for physicians provides more detail.)

I'm Not a Natural at Interacting with Patients (Unspoken: I'm Kind of a Nerd)

Some physicians were born with the ability to relate well with patients, and yes, they do have an advantage. But I've worked with many others who evolved from Dr. Aloof or Dr. Awkward to Dr. Personable because they worked at it.

Responses

- As much as relating to patients is an art, it is also a science. An interaction can be broken into key parts that should occur pretty much every time. These components can be learned—practiced, improved on, and eventually mastered.
- The single biggest factor that will help you relate to your patients is simply being mindful of the importance of each interaction. In other words, just thinking about it will improve performance. (Consider what happened in the First Physician Corporation case study presented in Chapter 1—scores began to improve when the group had only just begun to talk about the issue, raising awareness.)
- Over time, the strategies involved will become internalized and a natural part of your routine.

I'm Too Busy to Focus on This—I'm Overloaded

The problem here is overcoming the daily "whirlwind"—the overwhelming crush of issues and tasks physicians deal with just to get through a normal workday. The whirlwind sucks up every available minute, leaving zero time to focus on improving.

Responses

- Choose one thing. (When I coach doctors, I try to diagnose the *single biggest opportunity* they have to improve their interactions with patients. If the doctor agrees, we identify the *one thing* the doctor can do differently to seize that opportunity, and that's the only thing she works on until she does it every time without thinking about it—see Chapter 5.)

- I've found that if you focus on one very important thing, you can make it happen even inside the whirlwind. It may take weeks or a month to master it, but it will happen. Then you can turn to the next most impactful change that can be made. And so on. Be careful not to "pile on" suggestions for improvement in the face of the whirlwind. Over time, "one very important thing" each month becomes many very important things cumulatively—all of which have gradually become second nature.

Why Pick on Me? We Have Bigger Issues than This. The People at the Front Desk Are Rude!

Deflection and blame are so hardwired into human nature that this objection gets raised often. Fortunately, it's among the easiest to address.

Responses

- I won't argue with you on that, but that's not why you and I are talking today. Those front desk people are working on their issues. (They are, right?) Our office can work on more than one issue at the same time, especially when they involve different groups of people.
- Remember, it's the doctor whose interaction with the patient trumps all other experiences during the visit. Your efforts are the most important to patient satisfaction.
- We're not asking you to be so incredible that a patient's interaction with you dissolves their dissatisfaction with other aspects of our system. We're just asking you to do a good job with *your* interaction with the patient. That's all, and that's something that you can control.

Clinical Care Is My Priority

This is the noblest of objections, but it still poses a barrier to providing the best possible care and being "my wonderful doctor" in the eyes of the patient.

I encourage physician groups to have a dialogue about "how they keep score" (see Chapter 3). The healthiest groups balance multiple priorities, such as providing good clinical care, treating patients (and other members of the team) right, and being productive.

The key is to understand that several priorities always merit our attention.

Responses

- Providing good technical care is very important, but other things are important, too. Doctors who are exceptional clinicians sometimes lose patients to other (not nearly as technically skilled) providers who are more pleasant to deal with.

- The doctor–patient relationship is intimate, in its way, and involves caring not only for the body but for the soul, mind, and spirit. So the "soft" elements of care are very important, such as anticipating questions before they're even asked, helping patients make sense of complicated information, and putting them at ease.

- Patients who have good relationships with their doctors don't want to disappoint them. This regard leads to greater compliance, which leads to better clinical outcomes. It's all related.

So now you've countered your doctors' pesky objections and convinced them to pay attention to patient satisfaction. What's next? Helping them figure out what to do differently?

Not yet. First you need to understand why knowing what to do is, by itself, useless.

CHAPTER 5

How Physicians Can Make and Sustain Individual Behavior Changes

WHEN I COACH physicians to address their challenges, some make and sustain improvement. But others don't.

Why?

Because physicians are just people. And while most of us would say that becoming intentionally better at patient interactions is the right thing to do, it's also—for some physicians—a new behavior. And just like quitting smoking or losing weight, any new behavior can be tough to adopt and stick to.

The most frequent request I get from physician groups is "just tell us how to have great interactions with patients." And for years I gave lots of talks about key "make or break" elements of a typical patient interaction.

Unfortunately, those talks alone rarely led to improvements. Even after individual coaching had been completed, the following conversation occurred too frequently:

Bo (to a client several months later): "Have you been able to make that one key change we talked about?"

Physician: "No, but I'll start working on it soon. Really. I promise." (Or, "Yes I have," as his nose begins to grow.)

At some point, the engagement is over, the consultant goes home, and success is up to the client. Whether *I* have made an impact depends on *their* follow-through. Leaders in healthcare organizations are in the same situation. Their success depends on people on the front line.

I understand that moving from a current state to any desired future state—even when you know *exactly* what that future state should look like—can be difficult. And doctors often face additional barriers:

- They're incredibly busy. The time and energy necessary for improving patient satisfaction scores are consumed by other urgent patient care issues (some of them life threatening).
- As high achievers, they often try to tackle too many changes at once and get overwhelmed.
- They expect results fast, so they become impatient and frustrated with how long it takes for their hard work to show up in improved patient satisfaction scores.

When I went looking for resources to help, I found that most focus on the "whats"—what physicians should do: sit down, make eye contact, don't interrupt, and so on. While the whats are important, I've come to believe the more helpful question is "how"—how can a doctor, or a whole group of them, successfully change behavior?

INSIGHTS FROM THE SCIENCE OF CHANGE AND IMPROVEMENT

Some clients did make changes quickly. So I studied what they did and how they did it to develop a practical model for the how—a model for *executing and sustaining* positive behavior changes that produce excellent interactions with patients.

This model incorporates my experiences with successful doctors all over the United States and wide-ranging research on change, improvement, and getting things done. It includes concepts from the following sources, which I'll summarize next, before we dive into their application to physician–patient interactions:

- Prochaska and DiClemente's Stages of Change
- Shewhart and Deming's Plan, Do, Study, Act (PDSA)
- FranklinCovey's *4 Disciplines of Execution*
- Baldrige Excellence Framework (Health Care)

Stages of Change

The Stages of Change model was developed by James Prochaska and Carlos DiClemente from research into how people go about quitting smoking (and changing other behaviors)—some successfully, others not (Prochaska and DiClemente 1983).

It identifies six stages in a successful change: pre-contemplation (including denial and unawareness), contemplation, preparation for change, action, maintenance, and relapse. Helpful insights from this research include the following:

- Change is a process, and one must go through all the stages. If you don't start at the beginning, you'll almost certainly fail. In other words, the act of preparing to make a change can prevent failure.
- Some people will remain unaware of why making a change is important even as many, or most, people around them fully understand that change is necessary.
- Personal change must come from internal motivation. It never comes from external influences.
- Help is needed to sustain a successful change.

- Relapse is to be expected. It does not mean failure, but it should be prepared for and can be successfully addressed.

It may be helpful to understand why learning to behave differently with patients is actually easier than quitting smoking or losing weight:

- Most patient interactions are short and finite—a five- to ten-minute exchange. Physiological addiction to nicotine is ongoing.
- Unlike the smoker, the physician can be surrounded by a planned-for, built-in support network that includes peers trying to make similar changes, input from an internal or external coach, and leaders who are providing frequent encouragement and support.
- While the person quitting smoking may wish to avoid a devastating long-term outcome (illness or death), he faces relatively few short-term penalties that could hasten a behavior change. The doctor, however, can face significant short- or medium-term consequences: loss of patient volume, embarrassment when poor performance becomes known to peers, a much-reduced bonus, or loss of employment.

In other words, the doctor should be more immediately motivated than the smoker to change behaviors. Often, it's the job of the leader to create an environment that helps the doctor become internally motivated.

Plan, Do, Study, Act

Walter Shewhart and his better-known protégé, W. Edwards Deming, introduced the concept of learning and improving not in a linear fashion, but in cycles that build on knowledge gained from previous cycles. Early versions of PDSA (or its later iteration, Plan, Do, Check, Act [Moen and Norman 2014]), known as the Deming Wheel, could be summarized as "Design it, make it, put it on the market, assess whether it works, redesign it, and start the process over again."

While well known, PDSA is underappreciated in its applicability to a broad range of management (and personal) challenges. Many—maybe even most—problems can be attacked by trying a solution, assessing whether it leads to improvement, taking stock of what you've learned, trying a different solution, and repeating the cycle.

Here are the key takeaways:

- Progress is not linear but occurs in cycles. It comes from thoughtful trial and error, and its execution takes dedication, discipline, and patience (stubbornness may also be helpful). Success is directly related to how long you're willing to keep trying.
- Because the process isn't linear, it never stops. The quest for improvement on a big goal is ongoing.
- Improvement can best be achieved systematically. It requires commitment to an important goal and commitment to sustaining an ongoing process to achieve that goal.
- *Here's a big key:* Empiricism is important. Data, observations, and feedback are crucial for identifying needed changes and building a knowledge base to guide and accelerate progress.

The 4 Disciplines of Execution

The 4 Disciplines of Execution (McChesney, Covey, and Huling 2012) provides a framework for getting things done *even in the face of the whirlwind*—the day-to-day work of the organization that sucks time away from focusing on improvement.

Key insights:

- The daily challenges of operating an organization will always conspire to consume the time that could be devoted to improvement. The urgent (which act on you) always win out against the important (which you are trying to act on). And in healthcare, it's not like the urgent aren't important.

- When it comes to goals, less is more. The fewer goals you have, the more likely you are to achieve them. Having one to three goals is ideal. A helpful quote from *The 4 Disciplines*: "How do you eat an elephant? One bite at a time."

- *Here's another big key:* Act on lead measures, not lag measures. A lag measure, like a doctor's patient satisfaction percentile ranking, is useful as a long-term success indicator but cannot be acted on directly. A lead measure, such as "I will always ask the patient if he has any more questions before I leave the room," can be acted on and improved—today.

- Create a compelling way to keep score. A good scorecard will balance lag measures and lead measures (this concept is discussed in more detail later in this chapter).

- Create a cadence of accountability. For example, schedule a weekly 20-minute meeting to discuss progress on the few key goals, actions taken that week, and actions planned for next week. Perhaps conduct a quarterly review of each doctor's satisfaction scores in front of peers.

Baldrige Excellence Framework

Ideas from the Baldrige Excellence Framework for healthcare (Baldrige Performance Excellence Program 2015) are also helpful. This performance excellence framework poses questions aimed at developing high-performing organizations.

The insights that follow come from the framework itself; from Baldrige best-practice research by John Griffith, LFACHE, professor (retired) in the Department of Health Management and Policy at the University of Michigan School of Public Health, and his colleagues (Griffith and White 2005); and from my own years of experience as a Baldrige examiner and team leader and as a former leader at a Malcolm Baldrige National Quality Award–recipient organization.

- Progress can be made and sustained, even after previous attempts have failed (sound familiar?).
- Improvements are usually the result of systematic and sustained efforts (another familiar concept).
- Periodically taking stock of strengths and opportunities for improvement (OFIs) is important, both to mark and celebrate progress and to recalibrate future priorities.
- *Here's one more big key:* Leadership plays an important role in setting and communicating priorities, ensuring that systematic approaches are followed, and establishing a culture of accountability.
- Holding the workforce accountable, through a performance management system aligned with the few most important goals, is a significant element of organizational performance improvement.
- Thoughtfully rewarding and recognizing progress sustains and accelerates the journey.

So now that we have a solid background in the science of change, it's time to apply it to the real world—*your* real world of physicians who are contending with too little time, heavy patient loads, and the other challenges that abound in healthcare.

MY FIVE-STAGE MODEL

To improve interactions with patients, physicians must

1. become aware that a positive physician–patient interaction is very important and that, most of the time, the doctor controls whether this happens;

2. thoughtfully take stock of how well they interact with patients and prepare to undertake changes to do it better;

3. commit to one key change, and keep trying it until they've mastered it;

4. commit to making a second key change, and then continue the process as more changes are attempted, mastered, and sustained; and

5. take stock of their progress on behaviors they've changed in order to recognize and celebrate those efforts, ensure they are sustained, and identify future opportunities.

While a doctor can use this model to make improvements all by himself, without assistance from his colleagues or the system around him (more on this in Chapter 6), progress will be much faster—*and can be made by more physicians in a group*—if the process is supported by others who understand and follow it (more on that at the end of this chapter).

I can imagine you thinking, "Well, of course," about this model. But actually doing it will require more than recognition of a sensible concept—keep reading. For each stage, I offer detailed strategies and tools to help leaders guide their physicians through the process.

Stage 1: Awareness, Engagement, and Openness to Change

The first challenge, and one of the biggest, is getting physicians to not just "show up" but truly engage on the topic of patient satisfaction.

I often encounter health system leaders who want to get right to the assessment and action stages when they still have physicians who are not yet engaged. It won't work. Organizations can help a doctor move toward engagement by providing facilitation and support—even requiring change as a condition of employment. But ultimately it's the doctor's choice. Will she engage and make changes, or not? Organization-wide efforts will always fail if the individual doctor hasn't embraced the need to improve.

My hospital and large-group clients are often frustrated when a few physicians seem unwilling to engage or when they give lip service, but no action, to the process. These doctors sit quietly as the group discusses patient satisfaction and assume that the topic will fade away as other, more urgent issues replace it (more on preventing this in Stage 5).

Prochaska and DiClemente (1983) note that everyone moves through the early pre-contemplation and contemplation stages of change at different rates. So having doctors who don't jump right to engagement is to be expected. Many of the balky ones can become engaged in time, especially if they have some help.

What Leaders Can Do at This Stage

1. Create the expectation that high performance is possible and necessary.

2. Provide help to prompt doctors to begin the journey, as discussed in Chapter 3. Here's a summary:

    -   To begin the dialogue, ask each doctor to consider the main ways he judges whether he's doing a good job. Is "patient perception" on this list?

    -   Invite the doctor to consider the different physician personality types as they relate to engagement and which one(s)—superstar, nerd, prima donna, the unaware, or workhorse—most closely fits him. Getting a doctor to reflect on this connection may make him more willing to engage on the issue.

    -   Share recent patient satisfaction performance data and unsolicited patient compliments and complaints.

    -   Use one-on-one discussions to stimulate thought, encourage self-assessment, and determine engagement level.

    -   Continue to engage all the doctors in the group. Identify those who are motivated, and move them to the next stage. Continue working on the unengaged, until either they see the light or you determine that another course of action is necessary (see item 3).

3. When necessary, make the tough call on how long to tolerate disinterest before introducing the topic of parting ways. Just bringing up this option may be all it takes to trigger a turnaround. Or not. In which case, wouldn't the group's other members be better off without their unengaged colleagues? (This is a sensitive topic. Chapter 3 gives it the full attention it deserves.)

Stage 2: Assessing, Learning, and Preparing to Change

This stage begins when a doctor says (and sincerely believes; lip service doesn't count), "I'm totally aware of how important the physician–patient interaction is, and I understand that I can make some changes to do it better. *But now what do I do about it?*"

What Leaders Can Do at This Stage

For doctors, this stage includes gathering information and learning about *what* behaviors to change and *how* to change them.

Leaders should make sure the doctors also examine the barriers to successful change so they can think through potential roadblocks in advance and how to overcome them. Common roadblocks include the following:

- Being too busy to focus on improving
- Having a difficult time hiding frustration from difficult patients or families
- Language barriers

Still, it's helpful at this stage to also let doctors jump backward a bit and focus some of their thinking on the more black-and-white "whats"—*"What do I have to change to make the biggest improvement in my interactions with patients?"*

You can provide three useful tools that help them reach the answers.

Tool 1: A Summary of Feedback from Bo's Clients

I've observed thousands of physician–patient interactions in my shadowing and coaching engagements. Exhibit 5.1 identifies dozens of specific, high-impact behavior-change opportunities grouped into broad areas that follow the chronology of a typical patient interaction. (My forthcoming book for physicians provides more detail.)

Exhibit 5.1: A Framework for Engaging Patients

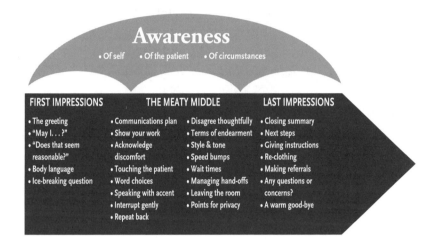

Tool 2: Self-Assessment

To help doctors prepare to change, I encourage leaders to offer a brief self-assessment tool, such as the one provided in the box on pages 75–78. This exercise prepares doctors for what's ahead and helps them identify changes that will make the biggest impact.

Tool 3: The Opinions of Others

Objective observers can provide valuable information to doctors. Observers can include the following:

- *A professional coach* (full disclosure: I am one) who shadows and observes individual physicians. It's the coach's job to identify strengths and challenges and communicate them supportively.

    A shadow coach observes doctor–patient interactions, taking note of how the patient is reacting, how the coach

Sample Self-Assessment for Physicians

Self-Assessment of Your Interactions with Patients

Instructions: This self-assessment relates to your interactions with your patients, and your patients' subsequent impressions of you. Don't take too much time to answer these questions. Usually your first impressions are the most accurate.

Which description best fits you?

_____ How my patients think about me is very important to me. I seem to be good at having positive interactions with them. I don't have to think about it—I'm a natural.

_____ How my patients think about me is very important to me. I have to put time, thought, and energy into having positive interactions with them.

_____ I don't think about my interactions with patients much, but I don't feel my interactions are perceived poorly. My main goal is to provide good clinical care.

_____ No one's ever thought of me as much of a "people person." My priority is to see a heavy case load each day and provide good clinical care.

If none of these descriptions hits the mark, jot down a sentence that more accurately describes your personal style in interacting with patients and where that fits in your professional priorities:

(continued)

(continued from previous page)

When it comes to interacting with patients, what are your greatest strengths? Limit your answers to a few of the biggest:

What one specific behavior could you change to most positively affect your patients' impressions of you? This is something you could either start doing or stop doing to make the biggest impact:

When answering the prior question, did you think of additional behaviors (two or three) that you could change to make an impact? What are they?

What do you see as the most significant barriers that might keep you from providing a better interaction with your patients?

(continued)

How do you think your patients rate your interactions with them?

_____ Much higher than most other providers in your specialty

_____ Somewhat higher than most other providers in your specialty

_____ About the same as other providers in your specialty

_____ Somewhat lower than most other providers in your specialty

_____ Much lower than most other providers in your specialty

If you have access to patient satisfaction survey data, what were your impressions of your most recent personal scores?

How often do you

- receive formal (written/e-mailed) thank-yous from satisfied patients? Have you noticed any themes among the comments?

- receive informal (verbal) thank-yous from satisfied patients? Any themes?

- receive formal (written or e-mailed) complaints from dissatisfied patients? Any themes?

(continued)

(continued from previous page)

[Leaders should add instructions that tell doctors what to do with their completed assessment. Options include

1. saving it to refer to later as they privately assess progress;

2. sharing it with peers at an upcoming staff meeting;

3. sharing it with the physician's leader in one-on-one discussion; or

4. combining the results with input from peers, coach, survey data, and other sources to create a complete picture of strengths and opportunities for improvement.]

would react if he were the patient, and how the coach might handle the situation if he were the doctor. Based on these observations, the coach provides individualized feedback on observed strengths and opportunities for improvement (OFIs).

- *An internal coach.* See Chapter 8 for an in-depth discussion on how to develop the shadow coaching capacity in your organization.

- *Staff.* Physicians can seek input from their nursing staff, medical assistants, or other caregivers who orbit them and observe their interactions with patients. I encourage doctors to (1) let their staff know why they're interested in getting feedback and why honesty is important to them and then (2) follow up with a paper survey, such as that provided in the box on pages 79–81, that staff can complete anonymously.

- *Colleagues.* The same approach as in the previous bullet point can be used if colleagues in a group typically observe each other interacting with patients.

- *And of course, patients.* Here I mean mining the "free text," verbatim feedback from patient satisfaction surveys as well as unsolicited notes of appreciation or complaint. (Some leading organizations are even putting comments like these online, for all to see. Refer to the box in Chapter 7, on pages 135–36, titled "Leverage Your Survey.")

Remember, the numeric scores tabulated at the end of a reporting period (often when the sample size becomes large enough to

---

Sample Staff/Peer Questionnaire

Request for Feedback on Interactions with Patients

To: My valued colleague

Would you please help me by providing some feedback? I would like to improve how I interact with patients to help our team earn higher satisfaction scores. I'm interested in your candid assessment of my strengths and weaknesses as I work with patients. **Note: Your feedback can be anonymous, if desired.**

By identifying my strengths, you'll help me reinforce what's already working. That positive feedback will help me maintain balance as I work on my opportunities for improvement—the areas where I most need to make changes.

My plan is to focus on one key opportunity at a time until I have mastered it. It may take some time to master each

(continued)

(continued from previous page)

one, but I'm committed to doing that once I prioritize the needed changes—based on feedback from you and others.

When you have completed this questionnaire, please put it in an envelope and place it in my mailbox.

1. When it comes to interacting with patients, what are my greatest strengths?

2. What one specific behavior could I change to most positively affect my patients' impressions of me? (This would be something I could start doing, stop doing, or do more consistently to make the biggest impact.)

3. Once I successfully address this one issue, what are one to three other behaviors I could change to positively affect my patients' impressions of me?

Going forward, I ask that you help me by:

- Occasionally asking me what I'm currently focused on to serve patients better. I intend to always be working on one important thing until I feel like I do it the right way every time without thinking about it. Your reminders will help me stay focused in our busy world.

- Letting me know whenever you feel I could have handled a situation with a patient better, or when you think I handled a situation exceptionally well.

(continued)

> - Letting me know whenever a patient compliments or critiques my behavior to you.
>
> *Thank you! I will truly appreciate your candid and constructive feedback and ongoing support.*
>
> From: _____ [physician requesting feedback] _____
>
> Date: _____
>
> You may include your name if you would like, but this is certainly not required: _____

permit a meaningful conclusion) are *lagging* indicators. They are very important but can't be influenced immediately or directly.

A more immediately helpful kind of patient feedback is provided by the verbatim survey comments (*leading* indicators, which can be acted on)—sometimes reported in batches but more suitably reported in real-time feedback that can be used for just-in-time service recovery. For example, when a patient reports, "Dr. Smith basically just walked out of the room when I clearly had unanswered questions," you now have excellent feedback for Dr. Smith to consider as he prioritizes his personal plan of action.

Sometimes patients give feedback even more directly. Occasionally they are brave enough to confront their doctor during or immediately after the visit, but more commonly they speak to a nurse or another staff member. Sometimes a complaint is relayed from a patient to a family member, who contacts another person on the care team or the hospital's patient relations department.

Leaders can help doctors see this feedback as invaluable as the doctors learn more about their personal opportunities to improve.

Stage 3: Making the Change

Now that the physician is ready to make the change, he must choose what to change and where to start. You can help him develop a game plan and understand what he's likely to experience as he proceeds. This plan includes

- identifying priorities;
- expecting and dealing with short-term failure and disappointment; and
- following the model to make the process manageable and, ultimately, successful.

Recall the insights from *The 4 Disciplines of Execution* (McChesney, Covey, and Huling 2012), one of which is to have *only a few important goals*. Having too many will cause doctors to lose focus, especially in the face of the whirlwind.

What Leaders Can Do at This Stage

As a coach, I help doctors consider information from their self-assessment, suggestions from others, and observations with patients to develop a prioritized list of strengths and OFIs (pronounced "oafies")—a concept borrowed from the Baldrige Excellence Framework. You can help them in much the same way.

First, Let Doctors Create Their Own (Short) List

Through shadowing and looking at patient feedback, I can often identify the one or two opportunities that will make the biggest impact for a physician. But it's more useful to work with each physician so that she *concurs* on which opportunities are most significant.

Physicians must own their prioritized lists before they can make headway on the top priority. Prochaska and DiClemente (1983) found that change must come from inside the person. The list can be changed to reflect what is learned later, but we're getting ahead of ourselves—that comes in Stage 5. For now, let's say:

> Dr. Smith has decided to improve how she makes a first impression on patients.

Second, Encourage the Doctors to Try a Change and See How It Works

Here we are applying Shewhart and Deming's PDSA cycle of learning and improvement in a simple but very focused way that has huge value.

The physician chooses a new behavior, tests it on her next patient—or a day's worth of patients—assesses how that test went, and then tweaks her approach.

> Dr. Smith commits to trying the following process with each patient: She will knock on the door. Then she will say warmly and respectfully, "Good morning, Mrs. Green, I'm Dr. Smith. I'm your physician today. Is this a good time for me to come in and see you?"

Third, Help Them Understand That Adjustments Are Expected

The key message for doctors (who are often impatient, perfectionistic, or both) is that things probably won't go perfectly the first time.

The first time a new behavior is tried, it will seem awkward. That's OK. Remember, PDSA is a cycle. You try something, you assess, you try something different, and you assess how well that went and what you learned.

> After some awkward pauses in the hallway, Dr. Smith sees that she should step into the patient's view before she starts speaking.

Fourth, Encourage and Expect Practice

Maybe different wording will make an interaction easier. Or different body language. But most often, it's repeated practice that makes a new behavior more comfortable.

The point is that doctors must practice the new behavior until it is perfected *and becomes second nature*. Then they must keep practicing it, being careful to note with each interaction whether it is being performed as desired.

> Dr. Smith has used her new way to make a good first impression for several weeks. She reports that it felt really weird at first. But through experimentation, repetition, and reflection, she has begun to feel comfortable using different wording that doesn't sound robotic. It has become natural for her.
>
> She decides to try adding a new line when appropriate: "May I pull up a chair so we can talk more comfortably?"
>
> After several more weeks of experimenting, Dr. Smith decides that she is very comfortable with her new skills at making a warm first impression. In fact, she notices that she does it without thinking about it. It's time for her to move on to her next opportunity for improvement: summarizing the main points of the interaction with the patient before departing.

(See Stage 4 for more on choosing what's next.)

How Long?

I often advise clients to work on one key priority for two to three weeks. Depending on the physician, the time to perfect a new behavior can be longer or shorter. It's usually not difficult to do something differently. What's hard is doing something differently *every time* without thinking about it.

An analogy is learning a new language and finally having a dream in that language for the first time. That's the level of familiarity one needs to reach before moving on to the next opportunity. And this always takes longer than a few practice runs.

The time frame also depends on the nature of the behavior that is being changed. Making a great first impression can be worked on with each new patient. But avoiding arguments with difficult patients will take longer to learn because those potential interactions happen less frequently.

What About a Broader Change?

A physician who has significant work to do on his interactions with patients can sometimes benefit from making a broader, more fundamental change—say, something like the following scenario:

> Before visiting every patient, I will pause and imagine that I am walking on stage to perform before 5,000 people, including the toughest critic from the *New York Times*. My goal is for the review in tomorrow's paper to be glowing.

I've seen a broad focus help doctors who chronically perform poorly with patients. They needed a first step to bring the issue of patient engagement to the front of their consciousness just prior to each encounter. Once that has occurred consistently, they begin to make other, more specific changes.

However, a broad change doesn't work for everybody. I've coached a few doctors who were so uncomfortable with change that we had to initially focus on a very simple and specific change, for example:

> I will look the patient in the eye and shake his hand when introducing myself.

Similarly, doctors who generally perform well with patients may benefit from only narrow, specific change opportunities because they already understand the big picture:

I will summarize the key points of our conversation before I say good-bye to help the patient remember *my* key points and so he knows I heard *his* key points.

The beauty of applying PDSA thinking is that it won't let you make a long-term mistake—you try something for a while, and then assess whether it's making a difference. Then you decide what to do next based on what you've learned.

Stage 4: Choosing the Next Change

Once a physician has implemented a change, has practiced it, and feels it has become second nature to her routine, it's time to choose the next change to make.

This process may be as simple as looking back at the prioritized list of opportunities developed back in Stage 2. If the doctor tried a broad approach for her first change (*"I will pause before each patient interaction and remember that connecting with this patient will be important to his health outcome"*), maybe she's ready to try a more targeted second change: *"I will not interrupt patients, even a little, until they have been talking for at least three minutes (unless it's absolutely necessary or they get totally off topic; then I'll redirect them as gently as I can)."*

Once the second change opportunity has been chosen, the physician can begin experimenting by practicing it with patients until she commands it. Then the next priority is chosen and the cycle continues.

What Leaders Can Do at This Stage
Keep checking in to make sure that (1) early efforts are eventually successful and (2) doctors don't rest on their laurels after early success. That first improvement should be followed by another and then another. This takes discipline on everyone's part.

Doctors—like the rest of us—are never "done" improving. But the process is tremendously rewarding, personally, professionally, financially—you name it. In my experience, doctors are energized by their first success and eager to continue.

Stage 5: Sustaining Each Change, and the Broader Journey

Organizations *must* intentionally support the latest successful small change a doctor makes as well as his longer-term journey toward improved interactions with patients. Otherwise, relapse is more likely to occur, and eventually the whole journey may be abandoned in the face of the daily whirlwind.

What Leaders Can Do at This Stage
Your job is to create ways to formally pause and take stock of progress and to formally reward improvement. Fortunately, efforts to sustain short-term gains and the longer-term journey are complementary, and they're neither difficult nor expensive to pursue. But they do require discipline.

Many of the tactics suggested below are group activities that can be supported by an organization, a practice group, or an employer. Some can be used by individual doctors who want to make progress on their own, even if their group or employer is not providing help. But, as emphasized earlier, progress will be accelerated if physicians have organizational support.

Daily/Weekly
Ongoing, frequent check-ins will help doctors keep the change they're currently working on at the top of their mind.

Many of my clients use *daily or weekly huddles* to quickly recap progress on key issues. I encourage this quick roundtable, in which physicians share their progress on individual changes—each talking for no more than 15 seconds. This is essentially a face-to-face version of the "confessionals" process used so successfully by First Physician Corporation (FPC) (see the case study in Chapter 1).

I also encourage the use of a *weekly journal or log*, in which each doctor keeps notes on progress and plans for future actions. Note-taking is especially important if team huddles aren't held. The tools for this type of check-in need not be cumbersome or complex. Its utility can be realized using a sheet of paper, sticky note, smartphone, or tablet in less than a minute.

Some doctors trade *weekly e-mails* with an appointed coach. The coach may be a colleague who's a superstar at patient interaction, in a buddy system. Or it may be another leader in the organization or an external person skilled at coaching on this subject. This practice hardwires a weekly reflection into their schedule, incorporates an opportunity to share progress and barriers, and injects both support and recommendations on how to best proceed through difficult periods when it seems like little progress is being made. This can take less than five minutes a week.

Also critical are *frequent reviews* to discuss any new, relevant data such as patient complaints or compliments received through formal processes (verbatim responses to the patient satisfaction survey) or informal feedback (e-mails or unsolicited notes of appreciation or complaint).

Monthly/Quarterly

I encourage physicians to take a deeper dive into their performance improvement progress several times each year. This process works best in a group, as doctors will benefit from learning from others and feel helpful peer pressure to prepare for the dialogue. Components include the following steps:

- *Reviewing patient satisfaction scores.* This review is ideally approached on an individual basis, but results can also be aggregated to share with the group as a whole. If the sample size is big enough, the data rarely lie (and they never lie over the long term), especially if they are compiled by an outside survey vendor. It's helpful to look at the data in two ways: in a time series to show improvement, and in comparison with peers or benchmarks to highlight achievement that others have accomplished.

- *Developing a personal action plan and scorecard* to maintain focus and track progress over the longer term. This step helps each physician be realistic about his movement toward improvement. Your job as a leader is to improve the odds that your physicians will do this by providing a template, survey results, and verbatim patient comments. A sample personal action plan and scorecard can be found in the box on pages 91–93.

As you look at these examples, note that I'm not a fan of rigidity in this area. I encourage clients to develop whatever format works for them. It might be as simple as a single-page, handwritten document. However, there *are* several elements I encourage including:

- A history of the individual physician's patient satisfaction scores, listed as a percentile
- The overall group patient satisfaction score
- The scores of all the other doctors in the group
- Recent unsolicited patient complaints or compliments with specific issues noted
- Specific, verbatim patient comments from satisfaction surveys
- A summary of the doctor's strengths
- A prioritized list of OFIs
- Which OFI is being worked on now
- Which OFIs have been converted to strengths and/or improved with past effort

Why is it worth the time to develop and update such materials? For doctors (and all of us), it is tremendously satisfying to track changes that have been made and sustained over a longer-term horizon. In addition, a scorecard or an action plan keeps the process active. It establishes and maintains focus. Each doctor is engaged in assessing his progress and where the next challenge lies. Although Kaoru Ishekawa, a Deming disciple, applied this quote in manufacturing, his point applies to patient satisfaction: "If standards and regulations are not revised in 6 months, it is proof that no one is seriously using them" (Moen and Norman 2014). I know an action plan is really being used if I see scribbles and coffee stains on it.

The scorecard or action plan balances short-term actions taken (leading indicators) with movement in

Sample Patient Satisfaction Scorecard and Action Plan

Patient Satisfaction Scorecard and Action Plan

For: _____Ben Smith_____

Time Period	My Percentile Score	The Group's Percentile Score	My Ranking in the Group
4th quarter	21st	59th	_7_ of _8_
1st quarter	38th	65th	_6_ of _8_
2nd quarter	70th	68th	_4_ of _8_
			_____ of _____
			_____ of _____
			_____ of _____

Strengths

I don't use medical jargon.

I make a good first impression. I'm comfortable introducing myself and making eye contact with patients.

I make a good last impression. I always leave by wishing them a good day or a "hope you feel better soon."

Opportunities for Improvement

I can be a little blunt with patients who disagree with my clinical judgment.

I interrupt patients to ask them questions and keep things moving.

(continued)

(continued from previous page)

I typically don't ask if they have questions. If they have a question, they can ask. I don't want to give them permission to keep me in the room longer than necessary.

Monthly Journal

Time Period	Actions and Observations
January	Just got our personal scores for the 1st time. Mine stink. Only Peter's are lower than mine. I've never thought much about the importance of my interactions with patients before. I just assumed I was doing OK. This is a wake-up call. I'm going to focus on the importance of a good interaction every time. Also being patient with rambling patients.
February	I'm letting patients talk for at least a minute before I interrupt. It's really hard when they're just rambling. Sometimes I just want to die!!!!! I got 2 patient complaints. One was from a patient with a crazy family. Marcus Welby couldn't have satisfied them. The other one was legit, in hindsight. We had differing opinions. My logic was on solid ground, but I think I came off like a jerk. I could have handled that better.
March	When they ramble, I play a game to see how I can diplomatically get them to keep moving. I'm getting better at this. I still try to remind myself before I go into the room that I haven't done a good job unless the patient is very satisfied with the way I treat them.

(continued)

April	Hey, my score improved to 38th percentile. I'm ahead of Sarah now. We started to buddy in a friendly competition to see who could improve the most. We e-mail each other every week with what we're focusing on. I'm working on asking to make sure the patient doesn't have any questions.
May	Still working on asking for questions. I got another complaint about arguing with a patient. The thing about this one was I knew I wasn't being at my best right after I argued with them. But I was tired and I moved on without apologizing. At least I now know when I'm entering the DANGER ZONE!!
June	Still asking for questions. Now also working on summarizing the conversation at the end. Funny thing. When I do that there seem to be fewer questions.
July	Scores are way up!!! 70th percentile!! I passed RJ and Philip. My scores are a little bit better than the group average! Still working on summarizing, asking for questions, and making sure I show the patient how I'm processing all the information to arrive at the best recommendation for what should happen next. I avoided a confrontation with one family who was looking for a fight!

patient satisfaction scores (a lagging indicator). If the needle isn't yet moving on the survey results, the doctor can find some satisfaction in his progress addressing opportunities as he interacts with patients day to day.

This tool also helps to sustain changes once they've been made. If a doctor gets so far as to work through all his OFIs, he can recalibrate—recycle former challenges already addressed back onto his priority list to make sure they are revisited and sustained.

- *Supplementing with other reporting mechanisms.* I have clients who require everyone in the group to report the personal improvement they're working on to the administrator every few months. One such client, FPC, summarized its confessionals into a report, which was e-mailed to everyone in the group. Other organizations do this via newsletters. (The administrator's current efforts toward improvement should be included, as well. More on this in Chapter 6.)

- *Providing formal rewards and recognition to each individual and to the whole group.* This step is vitally important. It will keep the faithful motivated. It will also encourage the stragglers to take the first steps past awareness to assessing, learning, and preparing to change.

  Recognition can be given for showing improvement on a lagging indicator:

  "Dr. Jones has reached the 50th percentile for overall patient satisfaction—a huge improvement!"

  "The group is now at the 50th percentile on patient satisfaction compared to similar groups in our specialty nationwide! Recall that as recently as last year we were consistently in the 20th to 25th percentile range. We have more ground to cover, but we can be proud of how far we've already come."

Recognition can also be given for improvement on a leading indicator:

> "Let's congratulate Dr. Sharma for mastering how to close every encounter by asking for questions and beginning to tackle how he gently, but firmly, deals with drug-seeking patients!"

It can even be given just for taking a next step in the process:

> "Dr. Park has completed a self-assessment and will be seeking input from some of you on her biggest opportunities to improve."

Don't forget to read aloud patients' notes of appreciation, especially if one is written to a physician who is struggling but trying hard.

Finally, let the physicians reward themselves and each other. Give them ample opportunities to relate personal reports of progress and milestones achieved and to receive observations from staff or colleagues. Praise from a colleague is one of the most powerful tools to reinforce behavior and motivate additional progress.

Annually/Ongoing

Several additional (very important) approaches help doctors sustain each change and will support their broader journey over time. I discuss two of these here.

Be sure to measure each individual physician's progress through your patient satisfaction survey. Consult with your patient satisfaction survey vendor to discuss strategies for gathering and reporting specific information for each physician. If it's too impractical or expensive, use patient complaint data and unsolicited compliments, which can often be ascribed to specific doctors.

This approach can be more difficult to pursue in specialties where teams of doctors care for a patient over an episode of care—hospitalists, for example. How do you know which physician is being assessed when the patient fills out the survey? It's easier to get specific data for each doctor for emergency medicine physicians and specialists who work in a clinic setting where one patient is seen by one doctor. However, it can be done within every specialty. I cover this strategy in more detail in Chapter 7.

Make sure physician engagement on this issue is embedded into annual accountability standards through the performance management system, if applicable, or through the credentialing process. This structure ensures that a formal review of how well a doctor handles interactions with patients will occur at scheduled intervals. Baldrige Award–recipient organizations report success in holding *each employee* accountable for focusing on one or two specific behaviors that will improve interactions with patients.

Now, take this one step further: The best healthcare organizations hold leaders accountable for patient satisfaction scores up the chain of command. Practice administrators are accountable, as are the hospital system leaders who manage those administrators. The system CEO should have concrete, measurable reasons to care about patient satisfaction in her organization's doctor offices, emergency departments, and nursing units. *Everyone should have some stake in the outcome.*

Use this model, and change will be achieved—and sustained. Time will pass, and you will assess the effectiveness of your new, improved system. You'll be able to make more changes. More improvement will occur. And the cycle will continue. How leaders go about building and improving a system that drives results is the focus of Chapter 6.

The Model Summarized, Plus Practical Action Steps

Stage 1: Awareness, engagement, and openness to change

- Raise awareness that this issue exists, and encourage engagement on the topic through one-on-one and group dialogue. Understand and communicate that everyone makes progress at his or her own pace but that *everyone* needs to engage at some point and begin to make progress.
- Have the discipline to not jump ahead in the process until you're ready.

Stage 2: Assessing, learning, and preparing to change

- Encourage self-assessment, and provide access to a self-assessment tool.
- Collect high-quality, provider-specific patient satisfaction and complaint and compliment data.
- Provide ideas on what to improve.
- Facilitate access to internal or external coaches.

Stage 3: Making the change

- Help doctors understand the importance of choosing just one thing to improve, how to practice that one thing, and how to continually reassess and learn from that experience.

Stage 4: Choosing the next change

- Encourage doctors to use input from a coach or an assessment tool to choose the next behavior to work on.

Stage 5: Sustaining each change, and the broader journey

- Facilitate access to high-performing colleagues as role models.

(continued)

(continued from previous page)

- Report progress and discuss barriers in the presence of peers.
- Meet regularly for ongoing dialogue and review: daily/ weekly huddles, monthly/quarterly review meetings, updates on patient satisfaction data compared to other groups in that specialty and among peers.
- Provide a template for a personal action plan and scorecard and continually supply relevant survey results and comments.
- Recognize and reward progress in the presence of peers.
- Embed performance on patient interactions into personal performance expectations in your organization's performance management system.

REFERENCES

Baldrige Performance Excellence Program. 2015. "Baldrige Excellence Framework." Updated February 4. www.nist.gov/baldrige/publications/hc_criteria.cfm.

Griffith, J. R., and K. R. White. 2005. "The Revolution in Hospital Management." *Journal of Healthcare Management* 50 (3): 170–89.

McChesney, C., S. Covey, and J. Huling. 2012. *The 4 Disciplines of Execution: Achieving Your Wildly Important Goals.* New York: Free Press.

Moen, R., and C. Norman. 2014. "Evolution of the PDCA Cycle." Accessed January 24. http://pkpinc.com/files/NA01MoenNormanFullpaper.pdf.

Prochaska, J. O., and C. C. DiClemente. 1983. "Stages and Processes of Self-Change of Smoking: Toward an Integrative Model of Change." *Journal of Consulting and Clinical Psychology* 51 (3): 390–95.

CHAPTER 6

How Leaders Can Ensure Success

"WE WISH OUR doctors could be more like your doctors," is what Brian Tsang, MD, president of First Physician Corporation (our case study, Chapter 1) often hears when he speaks to industry groups. The fact is, leaders can have tremendous influence on whether their physicians are like the high performers in Tsang's group.

If you're a health system CEO, a chief medical officer, a group practice administrator, a medical director, or anyone else responsible for the performance of a group of doctors, *your leadership matters.* Your efforts and approach to the challenge can have a huge impact on the individual and collective success of your physicians.

This isn't about your personal management style (that's another topic for another book). It's about building a *system* that produces improved results. Said another way, it's about putting the parts of a machine in place, many of which rely on other parts to operate in the most efficient and productive way.

Here's an example: Stanford Health Care, the academic health system affiliated with Stanford University, has used a wide array of integrated approaches to improve its physicians' patient satisfaction scores. According to Amir Dan Rubin, president and CEO (personal communication, November 5, 2014), the organization has accomplished this goal by

- making the right hires,
- setting expectations during the on-boarding process,
- providing coaching for doctors who need further support,
- tracking and reporting results,
- offering formal and informal rewards and recognition, and
- tying physician compensation to results.

Stanford's next initiative borrows a page from the consumer review website Yelp. It plans to place all patient satisfaction survey comments online, where anyone can search them by physician. This action creates unassailable transparency and very strong incentive for physicians to perform highly in this area.

Stanford's systematic approaches have paid off: Scores have risen from the 45th to the 95th percentile for inpatients, from the 10th to the 90th percentile in its cancer centers, and from the 15th to the 70th percentile in its outpatient clinics and medical group.

WHAT KIND OF LEADER ARE YOU?

Early in this book we talk about how you can help doctors assess how well they do with patients. I invite you to apply that concept to yourself—their leader—by introducing insights and questions you can use to assess how you (and the team you belong to) are leading.

The biggest question to ask yourself is,

> *What is the system I've put in place to allow the organization*
> *(or my corner of it) to accomplish the work it's trying to do?*

In *Built to Last,* Collins and Porras (2002) ask, "Are you a time teller or a clock builder?" Great leaders—clock builders—focus on creating systems that do the important work of the organization.

Time tellers, on the other hand, dive into the details, especially when a detail "becomes an issue."

Clock builders *create and improve* the system, while time tellers *are* the system.

Optimally, if your doctors' patient satisfaction scores are low, you will begin to methodically put some of the approaches from this book in place, especially from Chapters 3 and 5. You will begin to build a system—cog by cog—that gets doctors to grasp the issue, makes them accountable for their own scores, provides support for them as they begin to engage in changes to improve their performance, and responds when performance fails to meet expectations.

Again, optimally, you will try a new approach that is the most logical for your situation, let some time pass, and then assess how well it has worked. Then you'll tweak it, discontinue it, or continue it as is while adding a second approach that might improve results even more.

But the reality is that most of us aren't very systematic. Most of us jump to a new idea/tactic/program in reaction to an issue that has arisen. When that doesn't work, we switch gears and try something else. We're not thoughtful. We're not contemplative. We're under the gun and just want something—*anything*—to solve the problem we face today.

If this describes you or the leadership team you're part of, don't worry. You're still way ahead of the leaders who do little or nothing to address a problem or don't even understand that a problem exists.

BEING SYSTEMATIC IN AN UNDISCIPLINED ORGANIZATION

Frankly, I'm aware of many healthcare organizations that almost never take a systematic approach to managing themselves. This is especially true of the parts of those organizations that deliver services through physicians. And doubly so when they have just recently begun employing doctors or contracting with a third party to provide services that independent, community-based physicians had provided previously.

I'm not knocking the trend toward physician employment—after all, the Mayo Clinic, Henry Ford Health System, Kaiser Permanente, and Cleveland Clinic models produce exceptional results. But many new physician groups lack the organizational maturity of the Mayos of the world.

So, if you're a leader in a less mature organization or in one with many dysfunctions, and you don't have a hundred years to sort things out, what can you do to accelerate progress?

The rest of this chapter presents some of the key functions of a patient-centered system and key questions you might ask to keep progress moving. First, however, let's return to the concept of the clock builder.

Dedicate Eight Hours a Week to Being a Clock Builder

Here's the challenge I like to give leaders: Can you carve out 20 percent of your time to spend on assessing and improving your system to better meet the needs of your patients? That leaves 80 percent of your time to deal with legitimate crises, projects dumped on you at the last minute by your boss, urgent personnel issues, sitting in meetings you can't get out of, and so on. (Leaders also must perform some important *standard work* within that 80 percent of time. More on this at the end of the chapter.)

Use your eight hours a week to start seeing and managing the big picture:

- Can you draw or list on a large sheet of paper the parts of the system that you already have in place to achieve great patient satisfaction scores?
- Have you sat down with your physicians and talked about how each part of the system is performing—or not performing? You may be able to work with a few

thoughtful physicians in your group to figure out how to formalize the good things that are currently being done informally. Look for allies in this process.

- Figure out which part of the system is the highest priority for improving—and think about *how you determined that*.
- Identify what new tactic, approach, strategy, or model could be added to your system to create order and reliability out of chaos. (This book is filled with ideas.)

Be the Keeper of the Vision

Keeping patients top of mind is the best kind of "vision"—not that wordy statement in a frame in the lobby (although developing a concise one of those can be a good first step). I'm talking about formally establishing *caring for patients* as the Pole Star or the "beacon on the horizon" that guides all your efforts.

Vision is underappreciated and underused. Too often, leaders mistake vision for mere platitudes. Effective leaders leverage vision to help them with their heavy lifting and to keep everyone focused:

- Think of the vision as an elevator speech or a politician's brief stump speech to remind your team of what's most important, especially when other, less important topics conspire with human nature to overtake a patient-focused agenda.
- Reinforce the vision when you are talking with employees in huddles, when you're rounding, and when you're in staff meetings. As leader, you are the keeper of the vision. Communicating and reinforcing it should be a key part of your aforementioned standard work (see pages 127–29).
- Use the vision as a check question as you build the clock: "Does each part of our system make an *important contribution* to the achievement of our patient-focused vision?"

ELEVEN KEY COMPONENTS FOR YOUR PATIENT-CENTERED SYSTEM

To support the big picture—your vision of improved patient satisfaction—put 11 key components on your to-do list. Can you build them all at once? Of course not, but chances are good that you're already doing some of them informally in your organization. Formalize the activities that are already in place, prioritize the rest, start implementing or improving the one(s) with the most potential impact, and (very important!) periodically take a step back and assess how "the system" is performing. Then make more changes, and repeat.

1. Establish a Scorecard and Measures

A patient-centered vision is made more concrete by answering the question, "How will we know if we're doing a good job meeting our patients' needs?" You can begin to uncover the answer by developing and using a scorecard that includes specific measures of patients' perception of their care, such as the following:

- Patient satisfaction percentile ranking of the group (compared to peer groups)
- Number of providers in the group with patient satisfaction scores greater than the xth percentile, where x is the minimum level where intervention is not required
- Number of patient complaints filed with the patient relations department

Trend the measures across time, and compare results with peers when the data are available (and patient satisfaction survey data often are). The gold standard is to have very high scores on a percentile basis compared to similar provider groups.

2. Establish a Cadence for Reviewing Performance

A high-performing organization adheres to a schedule for reviewing its performance (for the organization or team as a whole; reviewing individuals' performance is a separate issue), and those reviews drive the organization's action agenda.

Toward this goal, I recommend sharing your scorecard measures with a cadence—on a schedule—that your organization is geared around. This rhythm will create discipline and help ensure that issues deserving action are those that will help you achieve your vision.

How to Build Accountability into Performance Reviews— a.k.a., Cascading the Heat

A colleague who is CEO of a hospital in a large system was telling me about his medical staff's patient satisfaction scores. They aren't good. In fact, improving patient satisfaction is a huge priority for his whole system—a priority that rivals even improving financial performance.

The individual hospitals' patient satisfaction results are reviewed and compared at quarterly meetings of all the CEOs at system headquarters. Leaders of the worst-performing hospitals are called out in front of their peers. "They catch some heat," my colleague says. And the expectation is clear: Fix the problem. As is often the case in meritocracies, exactly how to do that is left for each of them to figure out.

These CEOs are in a tough spot—with pressure from above and sitting many layers removed from the doctor–patient interaction. How do they get their doctors on board to

(continued)

(continued from previous page)

move the needle from "not so good" to at least "good enough to avoid embarrassment at the next quarterly meeting and the fear of being dismissed"?

I suggested to my friend that he and the other CEOs figure out how to "cascade the heat" downward to the physicians. Make *them* responsible for improving their scores. "If you let the heat stop with you, you're toast."

Easier said than done, right?

Right. But I'll pass along a strategy—and a few bonus ideas that work.

It starts with the data those CEOs were hammered with at the quarterly meetings. Show those numbers to the doctors! Let them see how poorly their performance compares with other hospitals in the system.

(If you're a stand-alone organization, show them how their data compare with your competitors, hospitals of similar sizes, etc.)

But that's not enough. You'll also have to make it personal. If you don't, each of them could blame her colleagues for the low collective score.

So drill down to individual physician patient satisfaction data.

Individual data are usually available from your survey vendor for doctors who care for patients who see only one provider during their episode of care (e.g., in the emergency department or physician office). It's trickier to

(continued)

obtain specific data for hospitalists and other doctors who serve inpatients seen by multiple doctors during their stay. To isolate scores for each doctor, you may have to ask your vendor to collect additional data on individual encounters during each patient's stay. I've also seen organizations do this through a special internal survey.

Trust me: This additional effort and expense is absolutely necessary and worth every cent. It may save your job.

Once you have the data for each doctor, you can replicate that uncomfortable meeting at headquarters. Put the data on the screen, showing the percentile rankings for each physician.

They will start to squirm, even if you don't name who's who at this point. Rank-order the scores from highest to lowest. Everyone will see that some physicians are doing magnificently and others not nearly so well.

Then come the magic words:

> In six months, we'll be showing the updated scores, but this time we'll have the names attached. We'll provide coaching and assistance to anyone who requests it, but it's up to you to improve your scores.

You won't need to say much more than that. You can rely on physicians' competitive nature and their aversion to being shamed in front of their peers to motivate changes in their behavior.

The other secret is to not let them forget about the approaching "reckoning" as day-to-day issues distract

(continued)

(continued from previous page)

them. Monthly reminders via e-mail and at meetings will keep the issue on the front burner.

Bonus Ideas for Cascading the Heat

- Set bonus pools for employed doctors based on individual (and perhaps also collective) improvement. Make the threshold for a payout fairly high—or at least require significant improvement among those starting in the cellar. Or establish a circuit breaker. Anyone with patient satisfaction scores below X is not eligible for a bonus, no matter how well they performed on other indicators.

- If the physicians are providing services through a contract with an independent group, the master contract should have patient satisfaction expectations embedded in it.

- Take each doctor's patient satisfaction scores into consideration when making schedules or assigning days off (and tell the physicians up front that you'll be doing that).

- Does someone have really poor scores after plenty of warnings? Don't renew his contract. And make sure everyone in the group knows why. This is a tough assignment, but one worth the discomfort. It will build credibility with the high performers and protect your team from having to "subsidize" the results of the poor performers in its collective scores.

- Move to include the quality of doctors' interactions with patients as a criterion for granting hospital privileges.

- And don't forget the most persuasive approach in the universe: public praise for those who have achieved and/or have sustained and/or are well on their way to significantly improved patient satisfaction scores. Doctors like gold stars, too.

Which of the following scenarios is most like how things operate in your organization?

> Look at the new patient satisfaction survey data from our vendor. There are some problematic trends in there. We'd better put this on the next provider meeting agenda when we have an opening. That might be two or three months out . . . .

or

> The November meeting is where we always discuss the third-quarter patient satisfaction survey data, come hell or high water. We receive those data from our vendor at the end of October. We have a schedule, and we stick to it whether the data are good, bad, or indifferent.

The schedule and the results of the performance data will help drive the priorities for change and determine what are considered "issues" in your organization. Needed changes won't be uncovered by happenstance or pushed forward in political power plays, and rarely will they be driven by emergencies.

3. Review Performance with an Eye Toward Action

As the team assesses each indicator on its scorecard, ask:

- Do we need to do something to help specific providers in the group (or maybe the whole group) get better?
- Can we say, "OK, nice job everyone, we're where we need to be"?
- Do we celebrate appropriately when we're doing a great job?

These kinds of questions should point to where you focus your actions.

It's critical that your review of performance indicators is active, not passive. Many organizations use a red/yellow/green color-coding system to simplify the review process—a shortcut made possible when thought has been given *in advance* to what performance level is acceptable for each indicator.

Indicators at acceptable levels (green) need no corrective action—but they might merit celebration. Those at marginally unacceptable levels (yellow) typically require a performance improvement effort to be implemented or at least readied in case results remain low in the next monitoring period. The red indicators need immediate attention.

When an indicator calls for follow-up to address unacceptable performance in patient satisfaction, it's often relatively easy to select an improvement tool to use. Recall from the case study in Chapter 1 that First Physician Corporation requires providers to be mentored for several hours (for which they are not paid) if their scores fall below the 75th percentile in any quarter.

Interventions for low scores that can be useful for any group include the following:

- General training for the entire team
- Coaching for selected individuals
- Peer mentoring for selected individuals
- Updating of self-assessments by selected individuals

Likewise, when performance improves or exceeds targets, the appropriate follow-up is to recognize and reinforce the performance through rewards, recognition, or celebrations. Leading organizations make a big deal out of good performance in a variety of ways, such as

- pizza parties for the whole team for favorable overall results,

- congratulatory handwritten notes,
- movie tickets for all team members,
- inclusion of all team members in a drawing for a big prize (an iPad, a weekend getaway, etc.), or
- special awards for individuals who have shown significant improvement.

To keep the rewards, recognition, and celebrations from getting stale, consider having a committee work on new ideas to keep them fresh and fun.

4. Use Performance Data to Incentivize Compensation

Of course, one very significant reward for improved performance is a larger paycheck. I strongly recommend using individual or group performance as a variable in determining how incentive bonus compensation is paid. In our case study, First Physician Corporation considered a formula that would award all members of the group the same amount on the basis of the overall group score. In other words, they would sink or swim together.

Some groups set the incentive compensation formula at the individual level—each doctor is rewarded, or not, based on his individual performance alone. Others blend individual and group performance: Before anyone can receive a bonus, the overall group performance must achieve a certain threshold. Once that threshold is reached, individual bonuses are determined by each doctor's own performance, with the highest-performing employees becoming eligible for the largest bonuses. It's likely that some employees won't get any bonus at all, which, one hopes, sends a strong message about the importance of patient satisfaction. If the group as a whole doesn't score highly enough, no one gets a bonus—even the highest individual performers—and that should send a strong message, too.

The key is to tie compensation for *every member of the team* to scorecard measures. Best-practice organizations define and communicate the payout formulas early in the year (or "evaluation period" if the bonuses are earned more frequently; I strongly suggest you consider this because they have more impact than only annual payouts) to have maximum influence on the behavior of each employee. Then they annually assess and modify the formula based on subsequent reviews of the system to most effectively incentivize performance. Ask, "Does our incentive compensation system best drive behaviors to get us the results we want to achieve?"

5. Attract and Retain Effective Team Members

In Chapter 3, I made the point that a group can raise its satisfaction scores if all team members improve their scores *or* if low-scoring providers are replaced by higher-scoring ones. All groups would be high scoring if only high performers were added to the team.

The best healthcare organizations screen prospective physicians for those who are good at interacting with patients. It's a threshold criterion for employment.

That means they don't hire candidates who clearly have problems engaging patients. Those organizations would rather leave a position open or fill it with a locum tenens than take someone they suspect will cause years of lower-than-tolerable patient satisfaction scores and a more-than-tolerable number of complaints (and who will require leaders to spend way too much time dealing with them).

But how can you tell? When I shadow and coach doctors who just don't get it, I ask their leaders if the signs were apparent during the hiring process. The response is always, "Yes, we saw the signs. But we were desperate to hire anybody with a medical license. We'd been searching for so long that we lowered our standards."

My advice is to be more systematic in the hiring process:

• Talk a lot about patient satisfaction in the interview to see how the candidates react.

- Ask them what they do to ensure a quality interaction with a patient. Do they have a thoughtful answer?
- Look to see if any patients have rated them online.
- Invite candidates to shadow one of your doctors—ostensibly so they can see "how you do things" in your group, but really to see how they interact with patients. Do they appear to enjoy it?
- Let them know that patient satisfaction scores are a key factor in bonus calculations. Note how they react.
- Check their references!

If you are disciplined in hiring and build a team of superstars, you'll find it will be easier to attract other high performers to your team.

6. Spend Time "Re-recruiting"

Retain your superstars by spending time with them. "Re-recruitment" is a formal process of reaching out individually to your high performers to let them know how much you appreciate their efforts.

The best leaders don't wait to do this until they catch wind that a provider might be looking to move on. Rather, they re-recruit proactively, on a well-considered cycle:

> February, June, and November are the months when I make the list of my highest performers and schedule brief sit-downs to let them know how much I appreciate their efforts and role-model performance. I probe for any issues that I can address that can help them become even more engaged or create a better work environment for them. I also follow up on any issues they raised with me the last time I met with them.

If you do this on a schedule, then you are a clock builder.

7. Deal with Low Performers

Low performers usually don't improve on their own. So the best organizations deal with them. And in healthcare organizations, this means dealing with problem doctors.

Embedding important measures from the scorecard into individual physicians' performance expectations drives accountability, prevents unpleasant surprises for the doctor, and makes the review process logical and objective. Objectivity is assured if you have collected a large enough patient satisfaction survey sample to gather statistically reliable results for each doctor.

It is hugely helpful to have a formal, written performance evaluation and improvement system in place so you aren't just making it up as you go. Most organizations have a formal performance review process; it's the "improvement" component that is too often left to chance.

If a doctor is clearly struggling, don't wait until the annual review to address the issue. Begin with an informal conversation. Offer support and resources. Progress to documented counseling, if necessary. Use a progressive disciplinary system next. And at the end of the process, don't be afraid to say, "It just isn't a good fit. We need to part ways." (For more on this, see Chapter 3.)

Though doctors are in short supply, high performers *can* be found and successfully recruited. And if you're smart about it, the next one you bring in will probably be better than the one you just had to let go.

8. Choose How You Listen to and Prioritize Physician Issues

It's impossible for leaders in healthcare organizations to *not* listen to physicians. The question is, how do you want to do it?

Do you like it when they catch you in the hall and complain to you? Maybe show up in your office unannounced and give you a piece of their mind? Or would you prefer a more systematic approach?

A CEO of a 400-bed hospital shared this story with me:

> My philosophy was to have an open-door policy—and that included physicians. But it got to the point where it just wasn't working. It was mostly talk therapy for the doctors without the problem ever getting solved. One day I finally snapped: "Doctor, you're here today with another issue. Do you know what I've done with the issue you dropped off yesterday? Do you see that pile of unaddressed physician issues sitting over there in the corner of my office? Here, let me throw today's issue on that pile just like I did with your issue from yesterday. I'll put it in there with the dozen issues other physicians dropped off this morning!"
>
> Now don't get me wrong. I'd really like to work on those issues. Really. But there are too many of them. And I'm getting pulled in a thousand different directions. And I feel really bad about it.
>
> We had to do something different because many of those issues weren't just pet peeves. To the contrary, many were significant problems. So I told my doctors, "You guys have to figure out which issues are the most important. Then we can assign them to teams—and I need you to serve on them—that can report back to the whole medical staff quarterly with progress."
>
> I put it on them to figure out the priorities. That did two things: One, it helped to guide us on where we focused our efforts. And two, whenever a doctor brought me a new issue, I could say, "You really need to take this one to the committee and see where it fits into the medical staff priorities."
>
> As it turned out, prioritizing the issues was a tough job. It took them six months to do it, and they almost killed each other! But they got it done, and we've made great progress since.

That organization developed a *system* to engage doctors and get their input on priorities for action.

Servant Leadership

Significantly, the CEO in the preceding example was acting as a *servant leader*. Taking this perspective when working with doctors often improves engagement and dialogue between you and members of the group. As a servant leader, your role is to serve the team. Your goals are to get people on board with the vision and remove barriers that stand in the way of their progress.

Servant leaders don't wait around to react to physician complaints. They actively seek out physicians' problems and manage solutions with a system. Servant leaders understand that frontline physicians are the main players—they have a key role in determining whether the organization will be successful. Servant leaders spend a lot of time making sure their employees have the opportunity to do well.

The box about reciprocity in Chapter 3 (see pages 51–53) offers a good example of servant leadership. In that situation, the leadership team correctly trusted that the orthopedic surgeons would become engaged when it worked on removing their barriers to success.

A final thought on listening to doctors: Leading organizations routinely use a *medical staff engagement survey*. You can take the survey results to physician meetings to report them transparently, to verify those results, and to ask your doctors to prioritize or re-prioritize the key issues if necessary. Good medical staff surveys are offered by several vendors.

To summarize this component of a patient-centered system, leading organizations have a system to engage and listen to doctors. The system works on a cadence, with certain activities happening throughout the year related to listening, confirming, prioritizing, and reporting progress (or lack thereof). Physicians are active participants at every step.

9. Make Patient Feedback Matter

It's human nature for physicians (or any employee, for that matter) to think about their needs more often than the needs of their customers (patients). And despite the fact that most caregivers truly care about their patients, few are entirely immune to placing their needs first, *especially if patient feedback is not clearly and routinely communicated to them.*

The parties who have a seat at the (staff meeting) table are often the ones best positioned to have their needs heard. (Ever had a meeting hijacked by a physician complaining about something that's driving her crazy?) It's the job of the leader to create a system that not only gets feedback from patients (merely the first and easiest step) but also puts that feedback in front of members of the team *and* makes sure the needs voiced in that feedback are clearly heard when priorities for improvement are identified and as decisions on subsequent actions are made.

Fortunately, getting feedback from patients is easy to do in the healthcare industry. Options discussed in other chapters include conducting a patient satisfaction survey and comparing its numeric scores to those of similar groups or organizations, reviewing the verbatim comments from the survey, and collecting unsolicited complaints and compliments from patients.

Sponsoring focus groups of past patients is another option. Many organizations use a third party for this revealing, small-group research. One approach is to partner with an expert from a local college or university to design and run the groups. Inviting only the patients of certain doctors most in need of feedback can be especially helpful. With patients' permission, noteworthy feedback can be recorded and shown to the providers most likely to benefit.

While getting feedback from patients is relatively easy, a more challenging task is to translate that feedback into a form easily digestible by physicians. The odds of success improve astronomically if you have built a system. You need

- a person who is in charge of making the raw survey data easily understandable,
- a template to present the information in a standard format (see the following box showing a sample PowerPoint presentation),
- a schedule for presenting the patient feedback to doctors detailing when and where this takes place and what happens if feedback is provided at a meeting that some doctors can't attend, and
- agreed-upon ways that the feedback will be followed up on.

With these pieces in place, you can be confident that the patient's viewpoint will be well represented on your work team's agenda.

Sample PowerPoint: XYZ Physician Group Patient Satisfaction Review—Key Information to Review Quarterly to Stay Focused

XYZ Physician Group
Patient Satisfaction Review
3rd Quarter

(continued)

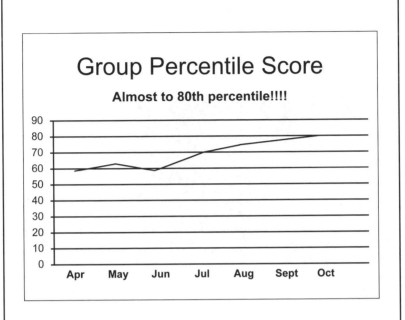

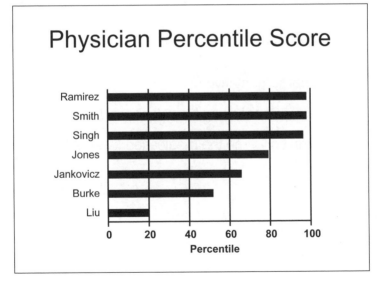

(continued)

(continued from previous page)

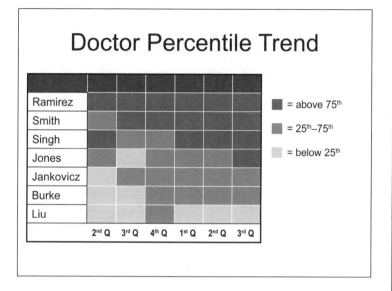

Doctor Percentile Trend

	2nd Q	3rd Q	4th Q	1st Q	2nd Q	3rd Q
Ramirez						
Smith						
Singh						
Jones						
Jankovicz						
Burke						
Liu						

■ = above 75th
■ = 25th–75th
☐ = below 25th

3rd Quarter Formal Complaints

- Rude/argumentative (3)

- Doctor was checking his cell phone (1)

- Wouldn't give me the medication I wanted (1)

(continued)

3rd Quarter Feedback from Surveys
Representative Examples—Criticisms

- ". . . doctor seemed rushed . . ."
- "He took a call during our visit."
- "He left before I could ask my question. It's not that I'm slow, but I had to formulate my question. He blew out of the room before I could get my thoughts together. I was embarrassed to ask him to wait."
- "I never felt like I got a good explanation of what was causing my pain."
- "She wasn't too interested in what I had to say. I felt like she jumped to conclusions. They didn't all make sense based on what I had been experiencing. I might want to try a different doctor next time."

3rd Quarter Feedback from Surveys
Representative Examples—Kudos!

- "Doctor Singh is so nice. I just love him."
- "I know I'm a rambler. But Dr. Smith is so diplomatic when I get off track."
- "Dr. Ramirez knows I don't like to take medications if I can avoid them. He did a nice job explaining options and why going on the medication was a very good idea."
- "The doctor did a nice job explaining everything. He really listened to everything I told him and took it all into account."
- "Dr. Jankovicz is really a kind person. She always asks me about my grandkids."

(continued)

(continued from previous page)

Lightning Roundtable

In 30 seconds or less, share with the group the behavior you're currently working on to improve:

Deep Dive Topic

Today's deep dive is sharing strategies to redirect patients who want to share their life story with you when you've got a very busy schedule in front of you.

- Offer something that has worked for you
- Total time limit: Five minutes
- Decide on next quarter's deep dive topic

10. Invest in Meaningful Education for Doctors

Much of this book is about helping doctors "up their game" in relating with patients. This is really about investing in them. Do you "invest" as best you can—anecdotally and on the fly? Or have you built a system?

- At least once a year (but ideally quarterly or twice a year), do you formally and objectively assess individual performance, have dialogue with each physician, and use her input to help her prioritize opportunities for improvement?
- Do you have well-developed and vetted resources to provide support for learning and development, beyond just "Let's try to find a conference on patient satisfaction basics; I've got some money budgeted for that"?

Resources can include this book, a mentor or coach, and a self-assessment or staff/peer assessments.

How NOT to Hire a Coaching Consultant

We consultants know that clients hire us because they need help. Best case (and we love these clients), they lack expertise or just want to bring new energy and perspective to an issue. Sometimes they simply don't have the time to spend on it—we understand that reality.

But in the worst case, clients are avoiding an uncomfortable situation. Essentially, they're putting off the problem.

Projects are doomed when an organization brings in a hired gun so it feels like it has done something instead of

(continued)

(continued from previous page)

rolling up its sleeves and spending time on the follow-up—communicating, implementing, monitoring. That takes focus, stick-to-itiveness, and discipline.

No big news there, right? But many clients don't realize that **what matters even more than follow-up is *preparing to change*.** Doctors should be primed for change before the coach walks in the door.

To illustrate, here's an example of how not to hire a coach or consultant:

> A doctor is getting too many patient complaints and has really low patient satisfaction scores. His medical director sits him down and tells him they're going to bring in a coach for him. A month later the doctor spends a day being shadowed by the coach and getting some feedback—end of coaching.
>
> The doctor then proceeds with his busy life, and it's as if nothing happened. His boss asks how it went, and the doctor says "fine." Six months later, the boss sees that patient satisfaction scores have not improved. That coach must not have known what he was doing!

Here's a much more successful scenario:

> The medical director sits down with the doctor who has low scores and explains her concern. The most important part of the conversation is the medical director explaining that it's the doctor's responsibility to make improvements within a particular time frame—maybe six to nine months—and how he does it is up to

(continued)

him. (If the medical director doesn't know how to begin this discussion, some phone time with the consultant can help.)

The medical director explains that this meeting will be followed up every three months, and patient satisfaction scores, patient complaints, and the doctor's thoughts on his own progress will be monitored.

Resources—such as self-assessment, this book, and/ or coaching—are made available to help the doctor. He can choose to use any of these resources. Or not. If the doctor is open to feedback from an outsider, he can talk with several coaches to find one he thinks will be most helpful.

The doctor spends a day with the coach, who helps him identify strengths and prioritize opportunities for improvement. The doctor asks for and receives advice on how to modify his behavior to address his opportunities while sustaining his strengths. He's motivated because it's his responsibility to improve.

Note that he chose coaching. It wasn't forced on him. He stays in weekly e-mail contact with the coach to keep focused.

Three months later, when he sits down with his medical director, they see that complaints have reduced a little. They recognize that not enough surveys have been received yet to get an accurate measure of progress. That's OK, because most of their conversation focuses on the doctor telling his boss what he's doing differently now and how he feels about his progress.

(continued)

(continued from previous page)

At the six-month meeting, they see that patient complaints are near zero and patient satisfaction scores have increased by 40 percentile points. The doctor's new behaviors are now hardwired into his daily routine. He's feeling more confident and is ready to tackle new opportunities for improvement.

This doctor was successful because

- he clearly understood that he was accountable for improving within a certain time frame;
- he was given the freedom (and responsibility) to choose what changes to make and which resources to use; and
- when he chose coaching, he was encouraged to talk to candidates to assess their chemistry before selecting one.

If You Bring in a Coach

Key points to consider when talking with potential coaches:

- Is the personal chemistry there?
- Does the coach seem to view her role as helping the doctor succeed, as opposed to finding fault?
- Is the coach positive and fun to be with?
- Does she seem able to give frank feedback in a thoughtful, respectful, inspiring tone?
- Does she see her role as providing encouragement and support for the doctor, rather than "reporting weaknesses" to the doctor's boss?

(continued)

If you want the coach to work with a group of doctors instead of a single physician, sometimes it makes sense for the whole group to meet with her before making the decision to proceed. If the client organization will pay travel costs, some consultants will "interview" with groups while offering some general thoughts on how to improve. This is a low-cost and low-risk way to get some initial help, give the group a chance to ask questions, and allow the doctors to become comfortable with a potential coach before committing to this resource.

11. Adopt Standard Work for Yourself

The concept of standard work comes to us from Lean management principles (Barnas 2011). It says that there is a best way to do work to achieve specified results. The challenge in adopting a standard work scheme is twofold: identifying what the standard work is and having the discipline to adhere to it.

Standard work makes intuitive sense to most leaders as they consider the work of their frontline team members. But leaders often have a difficult time understanding how standard work might apply to their own jobs.

As it relates to helping doctors have better interactions with patients, your standard work as a leader might include the following:

- Daily/weekly standard work for leaders
  - Rounding on doctors
    - To increase mindfulness of having quality interactions with patients
    - To ask what one key behavior each doctor is trying to improve

- To recognize each doctor's strengths
- To share any compliments received from patients
- Rounding on patients
  - To ask for any compliments or concerns related to caregivers
  - To generally assess their experience with their care provider(s)
- Rounding on direct reports
- Recognizing doctors for patient compliments received through surveys
- Communicating complaints to doctors and providing on-the-spot coaching
- Attending caregiver huddles to reinforce the patient-centered vision and key priorities
- Monthly/quarterly standard work for leaders
  - Aggregating patient satisfaction and complaint data
  - Preparing performance data for the monthly/quarterly team meeting
  - Preparing the agenda for the monthly/quarterly team meeting
  - Conducting the team meeting and keeping it "on agenda"
  - Ensuring all agreed-upon interventions are deployed following the team meeting (Are people following up?)
  - Meeting one-on-one with each direct report to review performance
  - Coaching doctors with scores below the minimum required threshold
  - Interviewing/screening new physician candidates for the ability to interact well with patients
  - Orienting/on-boarding new physicians

- Identifying parts of the system that aren't performing well as targets for improvement
- Leading/sponsoring process improvement teams

Of course, other aspects of standard work would apply to matters much broader than helping doctors achieve better patient interactions—clinical quality, productivity, and contributing to a positive workplace environment, to name a few. But those are topics for other books.

IN A NUTSHELL

Leaders can have a huge impact on physicians' efforts to improve their patient satisfaction scores. More successful leaders tend to see themselves as clock builders, not time tellers. They methodically implement approaches and build systems that require and support high performance. They are disciplined and see much of their effort as standard work to be accomplished through the system they've built.

Think about how you spend your day. Do you spend enough time building and improving the system and on your standard work within your system (rounding, coaching, meeting preparation, etc.)? Earlier in the chapter, I challenged leaders to spend at least 20 percent of their time working as the architect and improver of their system. This chapter provides ideas for components to include in that system.

That leaves 80 percent of your time for other things. I encourage leaders to spend half of that on planned standard work within the system they've created. That leaves 40 percent for urgencies, interminable meetings scheduled by others, activities that are unscheduled but important, and activities of questionable importance that you just can't escape.

REFERENCES

Barnas, K. 2011. "ThedaCare's Business Performance System: Sustaining Continuous Daily Improvement Through Hospital Management in a Lean Environment." *Joint Commission Journal on Quality and Patient Safety* 37 (9): 387–99, AP1–AP8.

Collins, J. C., and J. I. Porras. 2002. *Built to Last: Successful Habits of Visionary Companies,* 3rd ed. New York: HarperCollins.

CHAPTER 7

Issues with "the Data"—Our Best Friend and (Sometimes) Worst Enemy

WE ALL KNOW that using data to measure patient satisfaction is crucial. Without it, you're facing an uphill struggle to improve. But data can also be a cause of great frustration. At times, data can even lead to decision making that is counterproductive to the greater good.

Let's take a look at some of the lessons I've learned from working with "the data."

DATA PROVIDE ACCOUNTABILITY LIKE NOTHING ELSE

Over the past decade, more provider groups have started investing in patient satisfaction survey data. But I still come across physician groups and other healthcare organizations that don't, or that invest only the bare minimum to meet HCAHPS or CG-CAHPS requirements. The only conclusion I can draw is that these organizations don't take patient satisfaction very seriously.

Consider the business adage: "What isn't measured isn't managed." Until a group invests in survey data, it really can't answer the question, "How are we doing on patient satisfaction?" Once a group invests in survey data, it can begin to be accountable for providing a positive patient interaction in a way it never could before. And survey data can raise awareness of the issue like no other resource can.

DATA FOR EVERY PROVIDER

As we noted in the case study in Chapter 1, First Physician Corporation was asked by the hospital it served to improve its patient satisfaction performance, which had consistently been below the 30th percentile. The doctors didn't push back or make excuses. They knew full well that they hadn't placed any emphasis on patient satisfaction; it was not a performance measure they were actively managing.

But the group did make one very important request: The hospital would need to invest in a larger and more frequent survey sampling so statistically valid data would be available *for each member* of the group at least several times per year. The group's president, Brian Tsang, MD, says (personal communication, November 5, 2014):

> I knew if we had the data specific to each doctor with a large enough sample size then no one could hide. Everyone would have to be accountable. The data would speak for itself.

Having the opportunity to invest in a measurement system that results in individual accountability on an important performance indicator is a rare and wonderful thing. Seize it! You can't do this for your nurses, medical assistants, or other clinicians, but you can for your doctors, and the benefits will far outweigh the costs.

Unfortunately, many physician groups rely on scores that merely average their physicians' performances into a group aggregate. The resulting scores are typically mediocre, even if many of the doctors in a group would call themselves good, patient-focused physicians. Which brings us to . . . .

UNSEATING FREE RIDERS

When it comes to measuring individual physicians' patient satisfaction scores, some specialties, such as emergency medicine, have an advantage in that each patient's episode of care usually occurs with a single physician. So when a patient rates satisfaction, he's giving a score for one doctor. Other specialties, such as hospital medicine, do not have this built-in advantage. When a hospitalized patient rates her physician care, she has no choice but to lump together impressions of all the hospitalists (plus many consulting physicians) she saw during her stay.

The challenge to overcome here is akin to what economists call the "free rider problem." It arises when individuals face little or no incentive to bear the cost for an action, preferring to wait and hope the cost (or work) is borne by others. Here's an example: The American Medical Association (AMA) lobbies for physician interests. Any doctor can free-ride because he will benefit from the AMA's efforts on all doctors' behalf whether or not he is a dues-paying AMA member.

When the only patient satisfaction score known is the overall group score, every doctor can claim he is doing a great job and is pulling his weight—it must be others who are pushing the score down. And it's impossible to empirically challenge those claims.

I've seen hospitalists reviewing mediocre patient satisfaction data turn their group meeting into a "Liars Club," with each doctor telling the others how hard she's worked on improving her interactions with patients. They could have benefited from one of Margaret Thatcher's great observations (about another topic, but it fits): "Socialism works until you run out of other people's money." Here's my adaptation:

All of you can claim you're working on improving your patient satisfaction scores until our collective score falls to the very bottom. Then no one can pretend.

At that point, a lot of patients have already paid a price. Armed with individual data, you can prevent this from happening in the future. Bottom line: There's nothing like the objectivity of physician-specific patient satisfaction scores to help focus the attention of a group's members on the issue.

(If you're in charge of a hospitalist group, don't despair. Revisit Chapter 3 for ways to address the challenges of group patient satisfaction data.)

WHEN IS A SAMPLE BIG ENOUGH?

I'm not a statistician, but I did survive the bio stats course on the way to a master's degree in health services administration. The number that keeps coming up as the minimum sample size if you wish to *begin* to have *some* confidence that what you're seeing is *approximating* the actual score of *all* patients served . . . is 30. But to be safe, seek guidance from your survey vendor.

There's a trade-off between having a higher survey sampling, or *n* (and thus having more reliable data), and timeliness. You can always wait longer to build a bigger *n* and report your results, but then your data are less timely.

I've worked with some provider groups that collect a high enough *n* only annually. So their data are lagging indicators—in the extreme—for tracking performance. I've also worked with groups that invest a lot in the surveys so they can have a large enough *n* for the whole group on a monthly basis and for each provider three or four times each year. These fortunate groups can use their data not only as a more timely indicator of performance but also to get quicker feedback on the impact of changes doctors make to improve.

My advice is to survey as extensively and as often as your budget will allow. But if you have to choose between frequency and having data specific to each doctor, choose the latter. The

Leverage Your Survey

If you're asking your patient satisfaction survey vendor to provide only numeric performance data, you're leaving a lot of information on the table. Fully engage your vendor as a partner to help you make changes that will produce higher performance in the future. Some of the most effective ways you can do this are discussed next.

Share the open-ended responses

Post positive patient comments in waiting rooms. Let patients see them; perhaps they will mention to their doctor that they saw the nice things others had to say about him. Review both the positive and negative comments at staff meetings and post them in break rooms. Post the positive comments verbatim; scrub any provider identifiers out of the negative ones.

Letting the team see the critical comments makes everyone aware of the opportunities for improvement. Letting everyone see who's doing a great job helps your superstars serve as mentors and role models. This practice also creates helpful peer pressure for caregivers who don't see their name associated with positive comments very often.

Give doctors timely, individualized feedback from the verbatim responses

Some survey vendors are able to immediately send a system-generated e-mail to a provider each time a patient notes an open-ended response about her. When vendors use telephone (not pen-and-paper) surveys, usually administered a day or two following the patient encounter, doctors can receive these e-mails so quickly that they can often recall the specific context of the interaction. This

(continued)

(continued from previous page)

feedback is more understandable, actionable, *and valuable.*
These e-mails also have the benefit of frequency, helping
providers maintain constant awareness of the importance
of their daily interactions with patients.

Consider taking responses public

Some organizations are pressing the envelope to get
maximum value from their surveys' open-ended responses.
Stanford Health Care is in the process of putting all its patient
survey comments online for the public to see (Chapter 6).
According to Amir Dan Rubin, president and CEO (personal
communication, November 5, 2014):

> Organizations like Healthgrades are inviting patients to
> comment on their doctors in public forums for everyone
> to review. This is going to happen whether we want it
> to or not. If we do it ourselves, patients and prospective
> patients will turn to us as the trusted resource for
> information. And we want them to do that.
>
> We have the added benefit of having the data come from a
> source we and our doctors trust and are familiar with. We
> have high expectations and an improvement mentality, so
> why wouldn't we be willing to make this data accessible?
> And knowing that the data will be public is a strong
> motivator to act in a way that will make it look good.

As we discuss in Chapter 6, it's important to note that putting
comments online for the public was a natural extension
of the system Stanford Health Care put in place to help
its physicians interact better with patients. They had been
working at this for a while. If your organization finds itself at
square one, it would be premature, and not recommended,
to put physician-specific comments online as a first step.

value of introducing individual accountability trumps the value of frequency.

BE WARY OF *ANY* SAMPLING DATA

Remember that whenever you're using sampling data (defined as a *subset* of the patients you served), sampling error can occur. The odds of significant sampling error drop as the sample size increases, but they never get to zero. Even if you have a sample of more than 30, the results you see may not reflect reality.

Here's what happened to one of my clients. I worked with a physician assistant who "got religion" on patient satisfaction. He changed a few of the ways he interacted with patients and raised his scores to around the 80th percentile. When his scores then unexpectedly dropped to the 35th percentile, he became distraught. That score was based on a sampling of just over 30, so it met the minimum sample size threshold. I looked at his results and talked with him to try to determine whether he had made a change to his routine that might explain this drop.

We found nothing. Though I didn't think he had slipped into old habits, I advised him to use this finding as an opportunity to self-assess and refocus his efforts on delivering a great patient experience. We decided we would take a fresh look at his patient satisfaction performance data the following quarter.

When we did, we discovered that his scores had returned to the 80th percentile. There was no obvious cause for the downward blip; sometimes lightning strikes. Maybe it was just his turn to serve a bunch of hyper-critical patients who were determined to give their provider a low score no matter what. This happens sometimes.

So always treat statistical sampling data with some caution, especially if the stakes are high. For example, if you are considering termination of a provider, you'll most certainly want to wait until you see a long-term pattern of evidence. And if you're tying patient satisfaction scores to bonuses (a practice I highly recommend), you'll need to be absolutely clear with your doctors ahead of time that the "score will rule." Even if a doctor's score drops inexplicably, or even if he missed the threshold for the highest bonus by just one percentile, there will be no ignoring the numbers. So that means doctors should aspire to scores *well above* the cutoff for the highest bonus if they want to insulate themselves from sampling error.

DON'T RELY *ONLY* ON THE DATA

Yes, a survey with sufficient sample size is the only nonanecdotal way to determine how an individual physician or a group is performing on patient satisfaction. But if you stop there, you're only getting part of the value your survey can provide.

Verbatim responses to a survey's open-ended questions are invaluable. Although they are anecdotal, they can provide specific guidance on ways to improve. They go into more detail than the closed-ended survey questions and can give doctors a true sense of the behaviors that are—and are not—appreciated by patients.

And don't overlook sources of feedback beyond the survey. Patient complaints and unsolicited compliments received in writing or through the patient relations department are similarly invaluable. Like open-ended responses on the patient surveys, they give specific examples of behaviors that either detract from or enhance a positive experience.

Complaints and compliments can also be viewed as a check-and-balance for the survey data. If the survey data seem to blip in an unexpected direction (and typically this is downward), take a look at patient complaints to see if they corroborate the unexpected results. Feedback from observations—provided by colleagues on the care team or an independent party such as a coach—can also verify survey results.

One Way CG-CAHPS Doesn't Go Far Enough

About two-thirds of the 32 questions on the CG-CAHPS survey ask about the patient experience (AHRQ 2011). (For background on CG-CAHPS, see Chapter 2.) "Patient experience" includes interactions with nurses and doctors as well as processes for getting an appointment, encounters with front desk staff in person or on the phone, and so on. While only three questions ask about the doctors, one of those is key, and it appears at the end of the survey:

On a scale of 0–10, how do you rate this doctor?

The methodology considers responses of 9 or 10 as favorable. Responses of 8 or lower count as unfavorable as CG-CAHPS inches toward determining reimbursement levels. Clearly, this is an important question.

Unfortunately, the survey doesn't ask patients the equally important follow-up question, which would provide more *actionable* information: *Why do you feel that way?*

Your job is to answer that unasked question, or to get each of your doctors to answer it, so you have information that can be put to work guiding improvement efforts. Consider one of the following options:

1. Your patient satisfaction survey vendor can help you design a survey that supplements the government's CG-CAHPS questions. That way, you can get specific information to help doctors prevent dissatisfaction for future patients.
2. You can use the assessments discussed in Chapter 5, peer feedback, and responses from the open-ended survey questions to identify specific opportunities.

WHY MARGINAL PERFORMERS
HOLD ALL THE CARDS

Looking at individual-provider patient satisfaction data within a group is eye-opening. You can quickly see how changes in individual performance affect the overall group score.

Almost every group has both strong and weak performers. The superstars can help to raise the group's scores only to a small, sometimes negligible, degree because they don't have much room to improve. The key is getting the poor performers to improve. Can they bring their scores up to at least average? Can the average performers bring their scores up to where the highest performers are?

Or, for the biggest group improvement, can several of the poor performers get things so figured out that they'll join the superstars? I've seen that happen. The answers to those questions will determine whether the group's overall score can improve dramatically or just a little.

And what happens if the poorest performers are *gone*? Consider the hypothetical physician group in Exhibit 7.1. These graphs show that huge strides can be made if a few low-scoring doctors either get religion and bring their scores up or leave the group (on their own or with encouragement).

One other observation I'll make here is that everyone does not need to be at the 99th percentile for the group to achieve 99th percentile overall performance. Nationally, nearly every group, even the highest-performing ones, have doctors who drag down the overall score. (If yours doesn't, you're golden!) Say you have a group whose doctors are all good, but not great. Maybe everyone is performing around the 75th percentile, with no one much lower. This group might have an overall score of 90th percentile performance just because it has no low performers.

Exhibit 7.1: Example of How a Group's Percentile Score Improves When Low Performers Are Removed

Using Individual Doctor Data
Patient Satisfaction vs. All Doctors in Specialty X Nationally

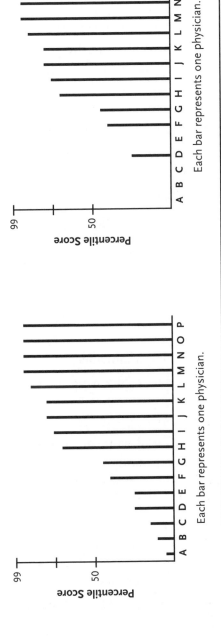

With Lowest Performers Present
Group patient satisfaction was about 60th percentile.

With Lowest Performers Gone
Group patient satisfaction rose to about 90th percentile.

Each bar represents one physician.

TO FOCUS ON SPECIFIC QUESTIONS OR NOT

I am often asked how important it is for doctors to focus on scores for specific survey questions versus focusing on their overall score. Most patient satisfaction surveys have questions that ask about the patient's perception of the physician in general, and often in specific ways, such as the following:

- Doctor was courteous.
- Doctor listened to what I had to say.
- Doctor was informative regarding my diagnosis and treatment.
- Doctor was concerned for my comfort.
- Doctor included me in my care.

The CG-CAHPS survey 2.0 includes many specific questions about the patient's perception of his interaction with the doctor. It concludes by asking the patient to rate the doctor on a 0–10 scale on two broad indicators (AHRQ 2011):

- Rating of provider
- Would recommend provider to family and friends

Most often, the overall score and scores for specific questions correlate. But if scores are low for a particular question, pay attention. It may shine a light on behaviors that can be changed or added to drive improvement.

If a doctor's scores on individual questions correlate within 25 percentile points of her overall score, counsel her to not fixate on the specifics. Suggest that she instead invest her time in an assessment, as discussed in Chapter 5, to identify specific changes that will lead to better interactions with patients (and scores on specific survey questions *may* serve as input to that assessment). As she successfully adopts those changes, she will see improvement in her overall scores and, generally, in her scores on the lower-scoring individual questions as well.

REFERENCE

Agency for Healthcare Research and Quality (AHRQ). 2011. "CAHPS® Clinician & Group Surveys, 12-Month Survey 2.0, Adult." Updated September 1. www.cahps.ahrq.gov/surveys-guidance/cg/instructions/12monthsurvey.html.

CHAPTER 8

How to Shadow Coach Physicians: A DIY Approach

I FREQUENTLY SHADOW coach physician clients. This activity has value for motivated doctors as a stand-alone activity, and it is especially powerful if offered as part of a broader system (discussed in Chapter 6) to help doctors improve patient interactions.

This chapter provides a road map for anyone (physician leader, practice manager, hospital administrator, etc.) who feels shadow coaching could be beneficial for doctors on the team but does not wish to turn to an outside expert.

A NOTE BEFORE WE GET STARTED

Often, an employer or practice leader mandates coaching for everyone in the group. If that includes a doctor who isn't open to the experience, you'll be wasting your time, and his. Attempting to shadow or coach a physician who doesn't want to participate is an exercise in futility.

Instead of plowing ahead against this resistance, take a step back for this particular doctor. Each physician travels his own path—first to the point of seeing the need to improve, then taking actions to do it. Chapters 3 and 4 will help you ease him down that path. And keep in mind that shadow coaching isn't always necessary if you can develop an improvement plan using other approaches.

WHY SHADOW COACHING IS SO POWERFUL

In my observations of thousands of physician–patient interactions, I have found that most doctors really enjoy being coached. They come away from it refreshed, recharged, and ready to improve further. Here's why:

- It's dedicated, private, one-on-one time. No colleagues or bosses are watching.
- The doctor can be open about what he sees as his strengths and weaknesses with patients.
- It provides time for individual questions and dialogue.
- Opportunities for improvement (OFIs) can be introduced in a diplomatic, tactful way with dialogue—so the physician is encouraged, rather than mandated, to buy in to the recommendations. Or he can suggest other OFIs and get the coach's feedback.
- Time can also be dedicated to highlighting and reinforcing individual strengths—an especially valuable part of the process. This helps energize the doctor for the journey ahead—tackling other challenges and converting them to strengths as well.
- It's individualized. The doctor doesn't have to waste time sitting through a group presentation of information that is too advanced, remedial, or inapplicable for his needs or style. His private session can focus completely on the basics if it needs to. Or it can focus on a few esoteric, high-level challenges if that fits better.

Here's an example. In my experience, of those physicians who try sitting down with the patient to improve interactions, about half will improve. For the other half, given their personal style, sitting down will make no difference. Why advise all doctors to sit when different advice will have more value for half of them? Any change is hard. You'll want to focus on the adjustments that add the most value for each individual doctor.

DO-IT-YOURSELF SHADOW COACHING

Having an internal person shadow and coach physicians delivers two big benefits. The first is cost savings. The second is avoiding a time-consuming process of selecting an outside coach who may or may not perform as advertised.

When considering whether to take the DIY approach, ask yourself:

- Is the internal person respected and credible to those being observed and coached?
- Is the person empathetic regarding patient needs and realistic regarding pressures faced by doctors?
- Can the person maintain a relationship of trust and not share the results with others?
- Can the person communicate OFIs in a tactful and helpful manner?
- Can the person engage in a dialogue with a doctor to come to agreement on the one or two key opportunities that most deserve attention before moving to others—that is, sift things down to the "vital few"?
- While your internal coach is getting acclimated to her role, will several physicians volunteer to be "guinea pigs"

while she gains experience and confidence as a coach?
And will you commit to continuing to offer this process,
so your organization can benefit from her growing
expertise?

- Can the person have fun and put people at ease? (This is
important!)

Obviously, mind-set and personality are paramount. If someone in your organization fits these characteristics, you've got a
good chance of being successful at DIY coaching.

The Goals of Shadow Coaching

To be the most effective observer and coach, keep the big picture
in mind. The doctor you're coaching is your client. Your job is to
provide feedback to help her improve, and to provide that feedback in a way that ensures it will actually be used.

Borrowing insights from my experiences as a Baldrige examiner,
the coach has three goals for every session with a client physician:

1. Highlight, acknowledge, and reinforce the client's
   strengths. Do this for all clients, even when their strengths
   are far outnumbered by their OFIs.

2. Recommend the one or two most impactful OFIs to
   improve interactions with patients. It's OK if the doctor
   identifies different opportunities. The goal is to get the
   doctor to buy in to making *some* single, significant change
   to start a journey of improvement.

3. Leave the physician with a renewed sense of commitment
   and motivation to stay focused on improving her
   interactions with patients (perhaps because you may return
   in a month or two to check on progress).

A little more on point 2: Here, less is more. Change is most sustainable when doctors tackle opportunities one at a time—allowing each change to become part of a new hardwired routine.

To take a concept from *The 4 Disciplines of Execution* model (McChesney, Covey, and Huling 2012), you'll want to identify and prioritize just a few of the most significant OFIs, so work can begin on each of them in order. Don't go overboard with the recommendations. The goal is to end the session with the client clearly focused on what her next steps are.

The Hawthorne Effect

Do doctors try to be on their best behavior because they know they're being watched? At least sometimes. This inclination is called the Hawthorne effect, based on research conducted decades ago at the Western Electric company, near Hawthorne, Illinois (Anteby and Khurana 2012).

The Hawthorne effect is one reason I always reinforce my clients' strengths as I review my observations with them. Even if they don't usually perform the positive behavior I observed (because they were minding their Ps and Qs for me), they will be encouraged to continue it if I recognize them for it.

You can also minimize the Hawthorne effect by being unobtrusive during observations and offering positive feedback while walking with the doctor between patient visits. As quickly as possible, you want the doctor to begin to see you as her trusted adviser, not someone she must impress.

Different Physicians Present Different Challenges

When I started shadow coaching physicians, it didn't take long to realize that they fall into a few major types, each presenting specific challenges to a coach. As their coach, you must be prepared to handle each group differently to provide the most helpful feedback to guide improvement.

Type 1: The Doctors Who Clearly "Get It"

Roughly a third of all physicians fall into this category. They achieve high patient satisfaction scores and rarely, if ever, receive a patient complaint. They interact with patients naturally and effectively. Paradoxically, they are often the doctors who think they need the most help, which may explain, in part, why they perform so well. They want to have a great relationship with every patient. They are hungry for feedback.

One challenge the coach faces with this type of doctor is that it can be difficult to quickly identify OFIs for them. However, nobody's perfect; small adjustments can almost always be made, as shown in the following section.

Advice for the Coach

Introduce these doctors to the concept of "trying to move 4s to 5s." In other words, their goal should be to have a perfect interaction every time. (Remember, this is a *goal*—something to work toward.) As you present this concept, give lots of supportive feedback on strengths, make sure they know that you think they're superstars, and ask them to serve as formal or informal role models for their colleagues. When patient satisfaction is being discussed in a group setting, it's important for the lowest scorers to hear that the high performers are working on improving, too:

> If Mary thinks she still needs to work on something— and everyone knows her patients love her—then maybe I should start working on something too. Maybe I can be more like her.

Focus on specific, discrete opportunities (which the doctors often identify themselves) related to patient interactions that happen infrequently but cause major challenges when they do. Examples are dealing with drug seekers or patients who have difficult family members and getting comfortable standing their ground while still being empathetic and retaining the patient's respect.

Consider recommending two opportunities that even high performers frequently miss:

- Complimenting other members of the care team when talking to the patient. For example, an emergency medicine doctor might say, *"My shift is over. My partner, Dr. Walton, will be taking over your care for me. He's an excellent doctor."* They should make this effort when they sincerely can (no faking it) and if possible when the complimented individual can hear them. It helps build the patient's confidence in the care team, and it supports a positive working environment for everyone.

- Summarizing the key points of the patient interaction at the end of the visit. This activity confirms to patients that their doctor heard what they said and increases the likelihood that they'll retain key information. Physicians are surprised when patients claim they weren't given information, because the physicians clearly gave it! But patients are often sick, tired, overwhelmed—and fallible. A closing summary makes the patient more likely to remember details and to give the doctor credit for "great communication."

Type 2: The "Regular Joes"

Members of this group are the easiest to coach because their opportunities are more obvious and are often easy to address once the individual is aware of them. The patient satisfaction scores of regular Joes typically range from a little above average to quite a bit below average. Still, this group possesses a balance of strengths and opportunities.

No specific challenges are inherent in this group beyond the always-present challenge: communicating opportunities in a non-threatening, non-offensive way so doctors buy into their OFIs, try a different approach to improvement, and stick with the process.

Advice for the Coach

When giving feedback to regular Joes, it's especially important to stress both strengths and opportunities. Don't jump right to the opportunities; build their confidence first by recognizing the behaviors they perform well.

Type 3: The Doctors Who Clearly Struggle

These are the 10–15 percent of doctors who have the lowest patient satisfaction survey scores. They probably also receive the most patient complaints. I instantly know I'm working with a doctor in this group when I hear him say or do something that makes me cringe.

Obviously, the OFIs for a struggling physician are many, so the first challenge is to help him sort out where to start. You must also help him gain confidence by pointing out his strengths, although these may be hard to identify.

Advice for the Coach

Sort out the OFIs and propose a short list of those that will have the greatest impact. It's important that your "client"—the doctor—buys into the list and the single behavior change at the top of that list: the place for him to begin.

Make sure the doctor understands the journey he is committing to and the realities of that journey. He should not expect perfection right away. Temporary setbacks are common—usually a result of getting very busy and becoming distracted from improving patient interactions.

Identify at least one strength to emphasize. Positive reinforcement will be incredibly powerful—even if the "strength" may be a real stretch or a behavior the doctor demonstrates less poorly than others. The key is to present this strength in a way that leaves the door open for further improvement in that area. If you can't come up with anything else, you can present as a strength something the doctor *didn't* do: *"I noticed you don't call patients 'Honey' or 'Dear.' That's great. I see doctors do that sometimes."*

Type 4: The Doctors Who Need Remedial Work

Sometimes physicians need extreme remediation in the area of patient interaction. For example, I've seen physicians just flat out tell patients in a negative tone that they were wrong. I've observed doctors get up and leave the patient's room with no explanation, though their conversation with the patient clearly was not over. Even more telling, these doctors didn't have any sense that what they did was problematic—and they knew I was watching!

Fewer than 5 percent of doctors have such major problems that someone in authority is thinking, "I'm not sure this doctor is worth it." However, they generate frequent patient and family complaints and receive patient satisfaction percentile scores in the low single digits, making their remediation (or termination) a top priority.

The first challenge in turning around a remedial-level physician is to get him to "see the light"; he places no value on what you're trying to do. The second is to determine where to start when a long list of behaviors must be addressed.

Advice for the Coach

The coach must be half "Dutch uncle" and half "horse whisperer." It's often necessary to be blunt but to mix that directness with humor (if possible) and supportive feedback so the physician will eventually trust the coach.

Remember, shadow coaching should be offered only to doctors who see value in it. With physicians of the remedial type, the coach may need to ask the question: *"Doctor, do you think our time together is resulting in any value for you?"*

If the physician seems unengaged, the coach should involve the physician's leader to consider a multiple-party conversation or try other, more basic approaches to help the physician engage (see Chapters 3 and 5).

Preparing Your Doctors for What Will Happen

Say you have decided to be the shadow coach or have selected a member of your team to serve as the coach. Here are some tips that will help you prepare your physicians for coaching.

I suggest two early, preparatory steps. One is to individually and informally ask each doctor whether she is looking forward to the experience, to get a feel for her frame of mind going in. Before the engagement gets too far along, you'll want to assess verbal and nonverbal cues for signs that a physician isn't supportive of the resources being provided for her benefit. Because you'll be working with doctors inside your own organization, you may already have a good sense of their predisposition toward coaching.

The other preparatory step is to have your doctors complete a brief self-assessment (see Chapter 5) in the days or weeks ahead of the coaching session. You'll want to review their self-assessments privately with each of them before observing any patient interactions. If a doctor hasn't completed the self-assessment, you can work through it with her collaboratively.

The key point is to get each doctor thinking about her self-identified strengths and opportunities and any special concerns or issues she would like you to be aware of. Remember, as coach you are working on behalf of the physician and should be flexible and responsive to special requests or other issues she raises.

Be sure to describe exactly how shadow coaching works and confirm that your doctors are comfortable with the process you will use as you work with them.

Don't overlook this point at the start: Make sure you both know how the physician will introduce you to the patients. It should be in a way that the doctor is comfortable with while being accurate, but brief. Patients usually won't be too curious about why you're with the doctor. I recommend your doctor saying something like, *"This is Mrs. Johnson. She is assisting me today."* At this point you smile, say hello, and shake the patient's hand if it seems appropriate.

Occasionally (perhaps one time out of ten) a patient will ask, "What are you assisting with?" or "Are you a doctor, too?" Your reply at that point should be honest but brief:

> I'm Dr. Smith's coach. I watch her work with patients and give her feedback on what she does well and what she might do differently to improve. She's very serious about providing good care and communication, and she's always interested in how she can do better.

Responses to this range from "OK" to "I had no idea doctors had coaches. That's great." From my experience, I can tell you that it will be rare that a patient would rather not have you in the room. However, you may occasionally wish to skip visits (by standing outside in the hall) if you think a patient is just too ill or excitable to have a third person present.

Also, make sure the doctor knows what you'll be doing after she introduces you: standing back and melting into the wall. You're in the room to observe. Your job is to say nothing and be as unobtrusive as possible. But don't keep a stone face. If the doctor or patient looks at you, smile, nod, and give nonverbal cues that you're interested in what they are saying to each other.

While Observing

On Taking Notes

I'm not a fan of taking lengthy notes while observing. It can be distracting for both doctor and patient. I do suggest carrying a small notepad on which you can occasionally scribble one or two words, especially if you can do so unobtrusively. This notation will likely be enough to tickle your memory after you leave the room and are making more extensive notes to communicate to the doctor later. However, you may want to wait to make even those briefest of notes until after you and the doctor have left the room.

Adopt Three Perspectives

It can be tricky to get the hang of this, but seeing the interaction from multiple points of view will help you develop better feedback for the physician.

1. *Reactions from the patient*—This perspective is the obvious one. Interpret the patient's questions and body language. Is the doctor connecting with her? Is clear two-way communication occurring? Is engagement evident? Later, when you're giving feedback to the doctor, your comments will be more credible if you can support them with examples: *"The patient didn't react favorably when you did/ said _____,"* or *"The patient really appreciated when you _____."*

2. *Reactions from the coach*—This point of view is less obvious as a source of feedback but is quite valuable. Patients don't always show how they feel. Sometimes you get no read from them. So the coach must mentally become a surrogate or stand-in for the average patient—and for the whole group of patients out there who are just like this patient. As I shadow coach, I note how *I* would have responded if I were the patient. (Interestingly, these observer-generated notes break about 50/50 into strengths and OFIs.)

3. *Reactions as if you were the doctor*—To gain this final perspective, I pretend I'm the doctor. How would I have gone about handling a specific situation? This technique can be useful in tricky, unique scenarios involving a difficult patient or family or in situations involving

drug-seeking or noncompliant patients who abuse substances or alcohol. Often, I play the role of doctor in my head as I'm assessing and replaying the exchange later.

Don't feel you need to always develop feedback from all three perspectives. Each provides value in different circumstances. When in doubt, the reaction from the patient is most significant. If you're not getting a reaction from the patient when you'd expect to, follow your gut and look at the exchange from the other two perspectives.

On Using a Checklist

I'm often asked if I work from a checklist when I observe, ticking off whether the physician "does this" or "doesn't do that." I do not use such a list, for several reasons. One is that I've been doing this so long that I've got it all in my head. The other (more important) reason is that the details of every physician–patient exchange are different. Doing, or not doing, certain things may or may not create a successful interaction with any single patient.

I never want my clients to feel like they're getting cookie-cutter feedback, and as their coach, you shouldn't either. I prefer to highlight areas where I feel a doctor really connected with the patient and areas where an exchange was unclear or confusing or when an opportunity was missed (or, at the extreme, when I cringed).

And the final reason I don't use a checklist is that it's distracting for the doctor and patient to see someone standing in the corner "keeping score" as their conversation proceeds.

What Is a Model Interaction?

Instead of a checklist, I recommend calling on a mental framework of a typical, successful patient–doctor exchange. See Exhibit 5.1 (in Chapter 5) for an example of what I use. Your framework may be simpler.

The key is to ask yourself several "bigger picture" questions related to *awareness* as you observe the doctor's performance relative to your framework.

Answering these questions will allow you to provide the most valuable feedback:

- Does the physician listen to what the patient is saying, and does the patient have confidence that he is actually being heard by the doctor?
- Does the patient understand what the physician is communicating?
- Is the doctor giving enough detail to allow the patient to gain a clear understanding of the situation?
- Is the doctor respectful of the patient?
- Does the physician show an awareness of the patient's needs—including needs that are unspoken or a need to explain things again or differently?

Pay attention to any behavior, gesture, or wording that makes you especially uncomfortable, and start thinking about how to diplomatically translate that discomfort to a teaching moment that will help the doctor. And on the flip side, make a mental note of anything that seems to make an especially positive impression on the patient or goes above and beyond the call of duty.

Between Each Patient Interaction

If, as I recommend, you do not take lengthy notes during each interaction, you'll want to take notes between visits, usually while the physician is working at the computer or talking with other members of the care team. You can write up what you've seen and begin to make some summary observations. As my coaching of a physician progresses, my notes grow from patient visit to patient visit, and I can begin to draw preliminary conclusions regarding her strengths and opportunities.

Huddle to Give Feedback

I always give verbal feedback to my clients in a brief huddle the same day I observe them, immediately after my observations are complete. My more formal follow-up occurs in the next day or two and includes the written Assessment and Action Plan, for the physician's eyes only. I e-mail the plan to the doctor directly. Samples are provided at the end of this chapter.

It's important to let doctors know ahead of time that this session will be brief and informal—a huddle, not a meeting or report—to avoid the potential apprehension that comes with such encounters.

The length of the huddle can vary. If I'm observing a number of relatively high-performing doctors and I'm moving quickly from one observation to the next, I might spend only 5 to 10 minutes with each physician. If I'm conducting day-long remedial coaching with a single physician, then an hour blocked off at the end of the day may be more appropriate. Much of that time will focus on basic education and helping the doctor focus on just one or two key behavior changes.

The goals of the huddle are to

- bring closure to what has happened during the day,
- offer encouragement and appreciation for what the physicians do and how they do it,
- let the doctors know I observed some positive things—and what those were, and
- get them thinking about one or two OFIs with the greatest potential impact and how those might be addressed.

Here are some important points to cover in the huddle:

- If the doctor is really struggling, start by showing him the framework you're using (again, I use Exhibit 5.1 in Chapter 5). This will help him see the big picture and grasp the components that are integral to a great physician–patient interaction. He can also see that your counsel is based on a well-considered model—it's not just random advice.
- Highlight at least one (but ideally several) observed strengths.
- Present one (or maybe two) of the biggest opportunities to be worked on. The doctor will probably recognize the wisdom of what you've presented. But if he has other ideas, discuss those. The key is to reach agreement to work on *something*. If he chooses a change that you see as having less of an impact, don't worry. Once he has successfully made one change, you can reintroduce the change you see as more important.
- The doctor is your client. At this early stage, his motivation to follow up after you've left him is more important than exactly what he's following up on.
- Suggest alternate ways to handle the opportunities that have been selected for improvement. Role-play to experiment with wording, if necessary (and if the doctor is comfortable doing this).
- Have the doctor go back and practice with a patient while you observe, if there's time (see the "Practice Changes" section following this list).
- Discuss how to continue to practice those changes and get them hardwired into the physician's routine.
- Encourage the doctor to continue the journey. Let him know the factors that drive doctors to successfully make changes and improve. In addition, acknowledge the typical

reasons some doctors who receive coaching don't follow through. This will demonstrate that you are realistic about the barriers that sometimes impede improvement.

- Discuss the resources and other support mechanisms available to him as he continues working on his opportunities (assuming your group or employer is providing support beyond the observing/coaching process).

Practice Changes

If time is available, huddle before the end of the day, discuss the most significant changes the doctor can make, agree on which one to tackle first, and then give him a chance to practice it with a few patients that same day in front of you.

This approach gives doctors confidence and allows the opportunity to get immediate feedback from you on their efforts. You can explain that the weird feeling they're having about doing something differently is normal—change always feels weird at first. This acknowledgment greatly increases the likelihood that the doctor will continue practicing the new behavior.

A FINAL WORD, AND A STORY

Let's recap the "hows" that we've covered in this book. Those are the approaches you and other leaders can use to engage your doctors and help them move forward with improving their interactions with patients and their resulting patient satisfaction scores:

- We've covered how to engage reluctant or unaware physicians and how to respond to specific objections they might raise (Chapters 3 and 4).

- We've delved deeply into the primary reason most physicians have trouble improving and given you a proven process that will help them make and sustain changes in their behavior (Chapter 5).
- We've talked about ways leaders can make perhaps the biggest difference—by building a system that both requires and supports high-quality physician–patient interactions (Chapter 6).
- We've told you how to deal with issues related to "the data" (Chapter 7) and how to personally coach individual physicians as they interact with patients (Chapter 8).

The concept that the quality of physician–patient interactions is ultimately a function of leadership can seem humbling, and even a little scary. I congratulate you for wading into this important topic. Assess your options for proceeding, and try a few things. After some time has passed, take a thoughtful pause to consider what you've learned, adjust, and proceed again.

As with most endeavors, the most important factor is to keep trying. Your success will be directly related to how long you're willing to stick with it.

Consider the experience of one of my clients, a small health system that had incurred financial penalties from Centers for Medicare & Medicaid Services on the basis of low HCAHPS scores.

The CEO and chief medical officer (CMO) knew that their employed hospitalists' abysmal patient satisfaction scores were a big problem. They had tried unsuccessfully to gain traction on the issue for several years.

These leaders knew that revealing doctor-specific scores might engage the physicians and move scores toward improvement, but they were scared. They have difficulty recruiting to their area and didn't want to alienate or lose any doctors.

So instead, they had "We really need to improve our scores" conversations. The doctors nodded and said they would. They had "Doctors should sit down when they see patients" conversations and even handed out an article about it. The doctors said they would sit down.

No changes in the scores.

So with nothing else working, the CEO and CMO finally got up the nerve to use the data. They told the doctors they were going to talk about patient satisfaction at the next meeting and hand out physician-specific scores. They even ordered a hot breakfast to increase attendance.

Meeting day arrived. Data were presented. And there were no fireworks. No one yelled "dirty pool." No one walked out. In fact, there wasn't much reaction or discussion at all. The meeting was—surprisingly and even disappointingly—anticlimactic.

But in the month following the meeting, one of the more recalcitrant doctors—who also had the very lowest scores—privately approached the CMO to take him up on his offer to help him improve. More doctors followed. At a staff meeting three months later, the physicians were sharing what they were each doing to improve their scores. Eighteen months after that, their scores—which had been in the teen-level percentiles—had risen to the 60th percentile.

"We still have a long way to go, but we're elated at how far we've come," the CMO says. "And our hospitalists are very proud of what they've achieved."

Sample Shadow Coaching Feedback Report for High Performer

**Physician Assessment and Action Plan
for Patient Satisfaction and Engagement Performance**

Physician Name: Mary Constantin*

Current patient satisfaction percentile score: 98th

Physician goal: Continue your exceptional interactions with patients. Become a role model within the group.

Action plan

Top priority: Continue to do the very polished and communicative things that you do to build excellent relationships with your patients and other members of the care team. See comments below for details.

Second priority: Be an active leader and role model in the group. Support your colleagues who aren't as good at satisfying patient interactions by talking about what you're working on to improve your own interactions with patients.

Third priority: Look for opportunities to compliment other members of the care team with your patients, whether these are nurses or your physician colleagues. This is "advanced advice" that I give only to the very highest performers. More details are provided in the comments below.

Comments from observations with patients:

- Observed an interaction with a female patient who was getting over flu-like symptoms. This was a model

*Fictional physician

(continued)

patient interaction. Your explanation was clear. You did a fantastic job summarizing your discussion before winding things down and saying good-bye. You asked if the patient had any questions—she did—and you were patient and took the time necessary to answer each one without seeming like you were busy and had to leave. You gave her the feeling that she could have talked to you all day. (I didn't see you give a business card to this patient, but I think you had seen her before, so you already knew each other.)

- Observed you interact with a female patient who had an infection in an arm and is also an IV drug user. You did a very nice job with her. You interviewed her to get her input on how she felt. You updated her on tests. You gave her your assessment of her overall progress. Once again, you summarized very well and made sure she knew when she would likely get discharged. You had great rapport with a patient who could have been a challenge.

- Observed you interact with a female patient who was nearing discharge in a day or two. You obviously had established an excellent relationship with her prior to this interaction. You used your sense of humor, which she really engaged with. I sense that you do a great job of "reading" your patients and interacting with them in a way that they respond to. You did a very nice job of letting the patient know before you began the physical exam (a very respectful practice that is appreciated by most patients).

- After spending time with you around other staff, it's clear they really like and respect you. I saw you use your sense of humor with them. And you create a comfortable environment for them to use their sense of humor with you.

- Observed you interact with a male patient who had cardiac issues. During your time with him, he apologized for interrupting you with a question. You replied, "That's

(continued)

(continued from previous page)

OK. This is a two-way conversation." That was wonderful to hear. You also ended the conversation by asking, "What else do we need to cover?"

Suggestions:

- Not much to say here because everything that I saw was quite good—"role model" to be more precise.

- Since I saw nothing in my shadowing that I would have done differently, you are receiving the type of suggestions that I give to really high performers:

  - Be an active leader and role model in the group. For example, when group members discuss what each is doing to improve, be sure to offer something that you're working on—even though you've already mastered most things. You want others thinking, "Mary is so good with her patients already and she's still working on things. I have no excuse to not have something I'm working on."

  - Look for opportunities to compliment other members of the care team with your patients, whether these are nurses or your physician colleagues. Patients like to see this. It makes them think more highly of everyone, including the giver of the compliment. And for maximum impact, sometimes give compliments when the person being complimented is within hearing distance. This builds a positive environment like few other behaviors can.

  - I often advise high performers to summarize the key points of the conversation with the patient along with next steps when wrapping up. Even high performers don't always do this. But you do! Keep up the good work.

Strengths:

- You really are a superstar at interacting with patients. See my detailed notes above about your interactions. I would only be duplicating my notes if I typed a list of strengths here.

Sample Shadow Coaching Feedback Report for Moderate Performer

Provider Action Plan and Assessment
for Patient Satisfaction and Engagement Performance

Provider Name: Will Delong**

Current patient satisfaction percentile score: 38th
Provider goal: Be at the 75th percentile in six to nine months. Then reassess your opportunities to improve and set a higher goal for 12 to 18 months out.
Action plan   *Top priority:* Keep doing all the things that you've been doing since you first saw your patient satisfaction scores last year and became motivated to move them higher.   *Second priority:* Work on your introduction. Try doing it a little slower to give the patient a chance to absorb meeting you and begin to establish rapport. More details are provided in the comments below.   *Third priority:* Try really hard not to interrupt patients when they're telling you their story. If they begin really drifting and you must interrupt, do it gently. See details in the comments below.   *Fourth priority:* Wrap up each encounter with a formal good-bye. Let the patient know you enjoyed meeting him and hope he feels better soon. (You'll use different words based on each situation. Use your judgment.) You might also ask one last time if your patient has any questions or if you can do anything else for him.

*Fictional physician   (continued)

(continued from previous page)

Self-assessment highlights:

- You have been completely displeased with your patient satisfaction scores since you first became aware of them last year, and you want them to be higher.
- You've been making adjustments to how you interact with patients to positively affect your scores.
- Your scores are up by 20 percentile points!
- You don't know what you should be doing differently to improve your scores further.

Comments from observations with patients:

- You're a fast talker. You're polite, but fast. I think the speed of your speech makes patients think you're rushing through your time with them. You can fix that with a few easy changes (more below).
- You introduced yourself nicely, albeit quickly.
- You frequently asked if the patient had any questions.
- You thoroughly explained to a patient "why" the prescribed pills are better than the over-the-counter cough syrup.
- Before questioning the patient, you gently broke the ice by asking, "What brings you in?" I'd like you to do that kind of ice breaking more frequently and focus on asking the question slowly.
- Before touching a patient, you said, "My hands are cold." This was good for two reasons: You warned the patient about your cold hands, and you warned the patient that you were about to touch her (always courteous). I recommend an additional step before touching a patient: Actually ask her if you may do a physical exam. They'll always say "yes," but they'll appreciate your asking permission and letting them participate in their care.

(continued)

- After explaining your plan for addressing the complaint, you asked the patient, "How does that plan sound?" Again, this allowed the patient to participate in his care. This was done very well. Try to do it more often, when appropriate.
- You were playful with your patients when appropriate, and you used your sense of humor. This connected you with your patients.

Suggestions:

- Keep doing all the things that you've been doing since you first saw your patient satisfaction scores last year and became motivated to move them higher! You've improved about 20 percentile points just by being more mindful of the importance of a good interaction.
- Work on your introduction. Try doing it a little slower to give the patient a chance to absorb the introduction and begin to build rapport. I noticed that you sped right through your introduction. You speak quickly, so it's important to get things started on the right foot and not give the impression that you want to get things over with quickly.
- I noticed that you often interrupted patients when they were telling you their story. Try really hard not to do that. If you just let them talk, you'll find they often answer your questions without prompting from you. If they begin really drifting and you must interrupt, do it gently.
- Wrap up each encounter with a formal good-bye. Let the patient know you enjoyed meeting him and hope he feels better soon. (You'll use different words based on each situation. Use your judgment.) You might also ask one last time if he has any questions or if you can do anything else for him. Because you work quickly, pausing briefly to say good-bye will prevent the patient from thinking you're cutting the visit short.

(continued)

(continued from previous page)

- Once you've mastered the suggestions above, try to do several important things I saw you do occasionally, but now do them every time:
  - When you recommend a specific course of action, make sure you ask the patient, "How does that sound?" (or something similar). This helps the patient think of the two of you as a team.
  - Let the patient see your logic in how you arrive at your clinical conclusion and next steps. I call this "thinking out loud." It gives the patient more trust in your clinical abilities.
  - Ask the patient's permission before touching him to do a physical exam. Patients notice when a doctor does this, and it shows that you respect them.

REFERENCES

Anteby, M., and R. Khurana. 2012. "A New Vision." Accessed April 15, 2015. www .library.hbs.edu/hc/hawthorne/anewvision.html.

McChesney, C., S. Covey, and J. Huling. 2012. *The 4 Disciplines of Execution: Achieving Your Wildly Important Goals.* New York: Free Press.

About the Author

Bo Snyder, FACHE, is a healthcare consultant, speaker, and coach. He splits his time between the C-suite, where he enjoys helping executives make decisions that have a big impact, and mentoring on the front line, where he is energized by doctors, nurses, and others who do the "real work" of our industry. Through shadowing and coaching, he supports their efforts to improve interactions with patients.

Snyder also helps healthcare organizations achieve better results by applying the Baldrige Excellence Framework. He volunteers his time as a Baldrige examiner at the national and state levels, and has led teams and site visits. He also frequently trains other examiners.

He began his career with Bronson Healthcare Group, in Kalamazoo, Michigan, serving in several administrative roles for 18 years. In his last few years with the organization, Snyder was deeply involved in efforts that led to Bronson's receipt of the Malcolm Baldrige National Quality Award in 2005. Inspired by the dramatic impact of the changes there, he formed his own consulting firm, Bo Snyder Consulting, Inc., to help other organizations similarly transform.

Snyder holds two degrees from the University of Michigan: from the Ross School of Business and from the Department of Health Management and Policy at the School of Public Health. He likes to remind people that Michigan has the number one–ranked health services management program in the country. And to help keep it there, he has served as the alumni board chair and mentors current students and recent graduates.

Snyder has a passionate (some say unhealthy) relationship with Michigan football and has missed only one game at the Big House since 1979.

THE AUTHOR WELCOMES YOUR FEEDBACK

One key point I make many times in this book is that to improve, one must get input on strengths and opportunities for improvement. With that information in hand, decisions on what and how to improve can be made.

I am willing to take my own advice.

Please contact me with comments or suggestions. I am most interested in the following:

- Areas of the book that are the most helpful to you
- Suggestions for changes or additions in future editions
- Your personal experiences that can add value to future editions, including volunteering your group to serve as a case study

You can find me at Bo@BoSnyderConsulting.com.